Hepatitis B Virus Antigens in Tissues

To
my wife Chhabi
and
my sons Jem and Raja

Hepatitis B Virus Antigens in Tissues

by **M.B.Ray** MBBS, PhD

Assistant Investigator
Department of Medical Investigation
Laboratory of Histochemistry and Cytochemistry
Catholic University of Leuven, Belgium

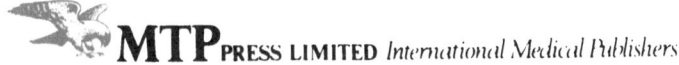**MTP**PRESS LIMITED *International Medical Publishers*

Published by
MTP Press Limited
Falcon House
Lancaster
England

British Library Cataloguing in Publication Data

Ray, M. B.
    Hepatitis B virus antigens in tissues.
    1. Hepatitis associated antigen
    I. Title
    616.3'623'0792   RC847

ISBN-13: 978-94-011-6237-1   e-ISBN-13: 978-94-011-6235-7
DOI: 10.1007/978-94-011-6235-7

Blackburn Times Press
Northgate
Blackburn, Lancs.
BB2 1AB

Contents

CONTENTS

vi

Foreword

Ever since the emergence of the concept of catharral jaundice by Virchow, viral hepatitis has eluded scientists as a pathogenetic enigma. A tremendous new impetus was given to hepatitis research by Baruch Blumberg's discovery of his 'Australia Antigen', now known as hepatitis B surface antigen. This led to an unheard-of outburst of research activity to elucidate the nature of the virus, its chemical and antigenic composition, its epidemiology, and pathogenetic mechanisms in the causation of liver disease. Coinciding with this period, modern medical science witnessed impressive progress in the analysis of the extraordinarily complex mechanism of immunological reactions. Immunohistochemical techniques for the detection of hepatitis B viral components are a product of this scientific progress in both areas. The application of such techniques forms the core of this work.

It represents a vast amount of work, performed during the course of several years, with meticulous application of advanced immunohistochemical techniques, combined with histopathology and clinical–pathological methods. This has resulted in the compilation of original results and new insights into the cellular and tissular localization of the antigenic components of the hepatitis B virus in different forms of chronic liver disease. The most outstanding results are the demonstration of the superior sensitivity of the applied immunohistochemical technique in the search for viral components in chronic hepatitis patients. and the differential distribution patterns of hepatitis B surface antigen in the various forms of chronic liver disease. Although the latter findings may not yet allow a complete understanding of viral replication and pathogenesis of liver cell damage in chronic hepatitis, it has been shown that they may serve as additional parameters in refining the diagnosis of the different forms of hepatitis B virus positive chronic liver disease.

In the last part of the work, an attempt is made to formulate a working hypothesis on the mechanism of liver cell necrosis, based on the original findings from the present work and on data from the literature. Even if the details of the presented hypothesis may have to be adjusted in the light of future work, one feels that the basic framework will remain, involving complex interactions of both humoral and cellular immune reactions in the pathogenesis of hepatic and of extrahepatic tissue damage. More importantly, the findings described in this work, some of them already confirmed by other workers, will remain established facts not to be ignored by any future attempts to reformulate a working hypothesis on the pathogenesis of hepatitis B virus positive acute and chronic liver disease.

What Dr M. B. Ray has achieved is an important step forward in the understanding of the pathogenesis of chronic hepatitis, which still remains one of the most enigmatic challenges of today's medical practice.

Leuven April 1979   Professor Dr V. Desmet

Preface

The past decade has been marked by a tremendous advance in the histopathological and immunological aspects of hepatitis research. The central stimulus was the discovery of hepatitis B virus antigen (Australia Antigen) by Dr B. S. Blumberg in 1964. The articles, reviews and progress reports written on hepatitis B are innumerable; these are devoted mostly to epidemiology and serological studies. This monograph, however, gives exclusive attention to the behaviour of the virus in different kinds of tissues, to the process of viral replication in the liver, to the transport of the virus from the cell to the circulation, to the host-defence mechanisms against it and to the process of development of clinical hepatitis.

The text includes both the published and unpublished material included in a thesis submitted in 1978 to the University of Leuven for the degree of Ph.D by the author.

The book is divided into four main parts. Commencing with a short historical review on the discovery of the hepatitis B antigen and its association with diseases, the first part deals with a detailed description of the various methods for the demonstration of hepatitis B virus antigens in tissues, followed by their evaluation and subsequent applications in clinical medicine for assessing patients with hepatitis B and hepatocellular carcinoma. The second part describes the sequence of appearance of hepatitis B virus components and associated immunopathological changes in experimental hepatitis B. It also analyses the effect of interferon on the distribution patterns of the viral products in blood and liver. The third part presents an increasingly important subject: extrahepatic manifestations in hepatitis B virus infection. The fourth part reviews the present state of knowledge in the field of immunobiology along with a new approach to the understanding of tissue damage in hepatitis B virus infection.

I would like to acknowledge my indebtedness to my teacher, Professor Dr V. Desmet who initiated my interest in liver disease. The present work owes much to his unfailing encouragement, advice and indispensable support. I am grateful to Professor Dr J. Degroote and Professor Dr J. Desmyter for allowing me to study their patients, biopsies and sera.

ix

PREFACE

Their help, advice and encouragement were invaluable to me. I specially thank Dr Fevery, Dr A. F. Bradburne and Dr Broekaert for their much needed cooperation.

I am most grateful to Professor R. N. M. MacSween, Department of Pathology, Western Infirmary, University of Glasgow, for his valuable remarks and suggestions in preparing this monograph.

I owe much to the help and cooperation of my colleagues and other staff members of this laboratory, in particular Dr C. Peeters, Dr B. van Damme and Dr R. de Vos. Special thanks are due to Dr R. de Vos for allowing me to use her electron microscopic data, and to Dr M. C. Kew, (Johannesburg) for the collaboration in the hepatocellular carcinoma work. It is indeed a pleasure to acknowledge Mrs M. Veulemans-Weckx, Mrs M. Vandenreyken-Bervoets and Mrs B. Tips-Smets for the huge amount of secretarial work needed in the preparation of this manuscript.

I thank Mr M. Rooseleers for his help in preparing the illustrations. I wish to thank the publishers and/or editors of the following journals for giving me permission to reproduce my published original material: *Journal of Immunological Methods* (Figures: 2.1A, 2.1B, 2.2A, 2.2B, 2.3, 2.4A, 2.4B); *Journal of Clinical Pathology* (Figure 3.3); *Gastroenterology* (Figures 2.11, 3.7, 4.1); *Clinical and Experimental Immunology* (Figures 5.1, 5.2, 5.3) and *The Lancet* (Chapter 8). Lastly, I deeply appreciate the support provided by the staff of the publisher, in particular Mr P. M. Lister, in preparing this monograph.

Leuven, April, 1979   M. B. Ray

Abbreviations

AHTC	acute hepatitis with signs of possible transition to chronicity
AMA	antimitochondrial antibodies
ANF	antinuclear factors
Anti-HBc	antibody to hepatitis B core antigen
Anti-HBe	antibody to hepatitis B e antigen
Anti-HBs	antibody to hepatitis B surface antigen
AusAb	radioimmunoassay kit (Abbott) containing materials for detection of antibody to hepatitis B surface antigen in blood
CAH	chronic aggressive hepatitis
CMI	cell mediated immunity
CPH	chronic persistent hepatitis
C-phase	core phase
DAB	diaminobenzidine
FITC	fluorescein isothiocynate
GAHu/C3/TRITC	goat immunoglobulin G against human complement component C3 conjugated with rhodamine
GAR/FITC/TRITC	goat antirabbit globulin conjugated with fluorescein or rhodamine
HBeAg	hepatitis B e antigen
HBV	hepatitis B virus
H & E	haematoxylin and eosin stain
HBsAg	hepatitis B surface antigen
HBcAg	hepatitis B core antigen
HCC	hepatocellular carcinoma
HLA	histocompatibility antigens
LMA	liver cell membrane auto-antibody
LSP	liver specific protein (antigen)

1

ABBREVIATIONS

PAP	peroxidase–antiperoxidase complexes
PAS	periodic acid Schiff reaction
PBS	phosphate buffered saline
PHA	phytohaemagglutinin
RAHu/C3/FITC	rabbit immunoglobulin G against human complement C3 conjugated with fluorescein
RAHu/IgG/FITC	rabbit antibody to human immunoglobulin G conjugated with fluoroescein
RIA	radioimmunoassay
SER	smooth endoplasmic reticulum
SMA	smooth muscle antibodies
S-phase	surface phase
SWAR/IgG	swine antibody to rabbit IgG
TRITC	tetramethyl rhodamine isothiocynate
VCF	*in vitro* complement fixation

General introduction – historical review

DISCOVERY OF AUSTRALIA ANTIGEN

The story of hepatitis B antigen began with an investigation of genetic differences in circulating low density lipoproteins. In the early 1960s, Dr B. S. Blumberg, a geneticist, began to evaluate the antigenic specificities of serum lipoprotein, which could be detected with sera of multiply transfused patients, e.g. in haemophiliacs who develop antibodies against certain lipoproteins (Blumberg *et al.*, 1962; Blumberg *et al.*, 1964). In

DISCOVERY OF AUSTRALIA ANTIGEN

(BLUMBERG AND COWORKERS – 1963)

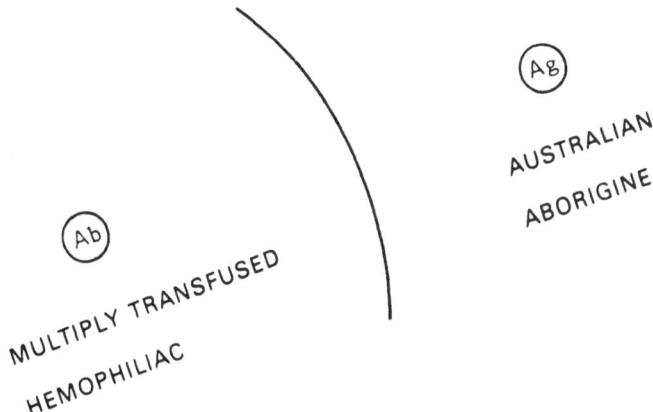

Figure 0.1 Diagramatic representation of Blumberg's discovery of hepatitis B antigen in Ouchterlony immunodiffusion agarose plate

3

1963, Blumberg (1964) tested sera from such patients for the presence of these antibodies by the Ouchterlony immunodiffusion technique. The panel of sera tested for the reaction with haemophilia sera included some obtained from foreign populations, one of which was from an Australian aborigine. This serum produced a precipitation reaction with sera from two haemophiliac patients which is shown diagramatically in Figure 0.1. Further study of the precipitin line showed that it differed from lipoproteins in that it stained only faintly with lipid stain but gave a strong reaction with protein stain. (Blumberg et al., 1965). Although the antigen was later found not to be especially common in Australian aborigines, it was given the tentative name 'Australia antigen'.

ASSOCIATION WITH HEPATITIS B

The first association between Australia antigen and disease was the discovery of its high prevalence in patients with acute leukaemia but general absence or very low incidence in normal Americans and in patients with other diseases (Blumberg et al., 1965). The antigen was later found to be sometimes present in patients with hepatitis (Blumberg et al., 1967).

In 1968, Prince (1968) reported an antigen present in the blood during the incubation period of serum hepatitis which was also identified by a precipitation reaction with sera from transfused patients. He named the antigen 'SH antigen'. As the frequency of SH antigen was higher in patients with serum hepatitis in comparison to that of normal blood donors, Prince suggested that the SH antigen represented circulating hepatitis viruses. This was the first firm link between the antigen and hepatitis, more specifically serum hepatitis.

In 1969, Gocke and Kavey (1969) reported an antigen in acute hepatitis, which reacted also with the sera from multiply transfused patients. Subsequent elaborate studies confirmed that the antigens identified by Blumberg, Prince and Gocke were identical.

In 1970, Blumberg et al. (1970) presented additional evidence that Australia antigen was closely associated with viral hepatitis. However, confusion arose from the fact that the antigen was found in subjects without signs of liver disease and in hepatitis patients without history of parenteral exposure. The problem was essentially solved by Krugman and co-workers (Krugman et al., 1967) by exposing volunteers to infectious material isolated from patients with two distinct types of hepatitis which they named MS_1 (short incubation hepatitis, hepatitis A) and MS_2 (long incubation hepatitis, hepatitis B).

Serum samples obtained during infection with MS_1 and MS_2 were examined for the presence of Australia antigen and SH antigen (Giles

4

et al., 1969). It was found that Australia antigen/SH antigen appeared exclusively in children infected with MS_2.

POLYMORPHISM OF HBV AND ASSOCIATED ANTIGENS

Viral structure and terminology

The nature of the hepatitis B antigens was determined by biophysical techniques and electron microscopy. The antigen can be purified by density gradient centrifugation (Gerin *et al.*, 1971). Electron microscopic examination of such purified material showed spherical particles of 22 nm in diameter and tubular forms sometimes over 100 nm in length. These particles do not contain nucleic acid. Subsequently, purified antigen obtained from patients with acute hepatitis was examined by Dane and co-workers (1970) and was found to contain an additional particle, 42 nm in diameter with a well defined coat on the surface and a core in the centre. This large particle is called the Dane particle and is generally thought to represent the hepatitis B virion (HBV). The structure and composition of HBV is schematically shown in Figure 0.2.

Antibody to Blumberg's Australia antigen reacts with the outer coat and not with the inner core of the Dane particle (Almeida *et al.*, 1971). A different antibody that reacts with the inner core has been found in the sera of patients with antigen positive hepatitis (Hoofnagle *et al.*, 1973).

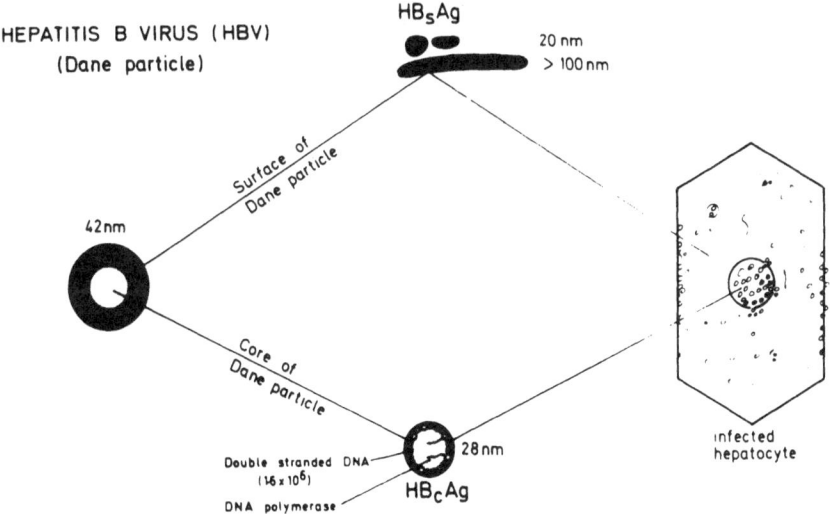

Figure 0.2 Schematic representation of the morphological forms of HBV antigens observed in blood and in hepatocytes

The identification of these two antigen systems led to a new nomenclature of the HBV antigens. The surface protein of the Dane particle and the major constituent of the spherical and tubular forms is termed hepatitis B surface antigen (HBsAg) and the core of the Dane particle is named hepatitis B core antigen (HBcAg). These two antigen systems can be identified by their respective antibodies, i.e. anti-HBs and anti-HBc.

Subtypes of HBsAg

HBsAg contains different subtypes, a group specific determinant a, and many additional mutually exclusive subdeterminant pairs, d–y and w–r. The w determinant also has mutually exclusive smaller subdeterminants. HBsAg positive sera can be divided mainly into four groups, adw, ayw, adr and ayr (Le Bouvier, 1972). These subtypes of HBsAg have been used as epidemiological markers but do not appear to have major clinical importance (Le Bouvier, 1973). Recently, however, infantile papular acro-dermatitis has been associated with HBsAg subtype ayw (Ishimaru *et al.*, 1976; Colombo *et al.*, 1977).

'e' Antigen (HBeAg)

In 1972, Magnius and Espmark described a soluble antigen different from the classical subtypes of HBsAg in the sera of patients with HBsAg positive hepatitis and named it 'e' antigen (Magnius and Espmark, 1972). The presence of HBeAg has been associated with active chronic hepatitis and with higher infectivity whereas its antibody, i.e. anti-HBe, is found mostly in healthy HBsAg carriers and rarely in acute and chronic hepatitis B (Nielson *et al.*, 1974).

Delta (δ) antigen

In 1977, Rizzetto and co-workers (Rizzetto *et al.*, 1977) described a new antigen in the hepatocytic nuclei of HBsAg associated hepatitis patients, named delta (δ) antigen, which has not yet been detected in the serum. By an indirect immunofluorescence technique delta antibody (anti-δ) was demonstrated in patients with δ antigen in the liver. Preliminary investi-gation shows that δ antigen and HBcAg are mutually exclusive. The clinical and immunopathological values of this new antigen–antibody system await further study.

Other components of HBV

Circular double-stranded DNA with a molecular weight of around 1×10^6 has been found in core particles isolated from infected human liver (Hirschman *et al.*, 1974a). The DNA isolated (mol. wt. 1.6×10^6) from

Dane particles is also found to be double-stranded (Overby *et al.*, 1975). A viral specific enzyme – DNA polymerase – has been identified in the Dane particle core (Kaplan *et al.*, 1973; Robinson and Greenman, 1974; Hirschman *et al.*, 1974b) and found to appear in the blood prior to clinical hepatitis (Krugman *et al.*, 1974). The exact site and mode of synthesis of viral DNA and DNA polymerase is still not clear. However, current evidence suggests that they may be synthesized in the hepatocytic cytoplasm (Hirschman, 1975). The details of viral replication are still obscure; hepatitis B virus seems to be an unusual type of DNA virus.

References

Almeida, J. D., Rubenstein, D. and Stott, E. J. (1971). New antigen–antibody system in Australia antigen positive hepatitis. *Lancet*, 2, 1225

Blumberg, B. S. (1964). Polymorphisms of serum proteins and the development of iso-precipetins in transfused patients. *Bull. N.Y. Acad Med.*, 40, 377

Blumberg, B. S., Dray, S. and Robinson, J. C. (1962). Antigen polymorphism of a low-density beta-lipoprotein. Allotypy in human serum. *Nature*, 194, 656

Blumberg, B. S., Alter, H. J., Riddell, N. M. and Erlandson, M. (1964). Multiple antigenic specificities of serum lipoproteins detected with sera of transfused patients. *Vox Sang.*, 9, 128

Blumberg, B. S., Alter, H. J. and Visnich, S. (1965). A new antigen in leukaemia sera. *JAMA*, 191, 541

Blumberg, B. S., Gerstley, B. J. S., Hungerford, D. A., London, W. T. and Sutnick, A. I. (1967). A serum antigen (Australia antigen) in Down's Syndrome, leukaemia and hepatitis. *Ann. Int. Med.*, 66, 924

Blumberg, B. S., Sutnick, A. I., London, W. T. and Millman, I. (1970). Current concept: Australia antigen and hepatitis. *N. Engl. J. Med.*, 283, 349

Colombo, M., Gerber, M. A., Vernace, S. J., Gianotti, F. and Paronetto, F. (1977). Immune response to hepatitis B virus in children with papular acrodermatitis. *Gastroenterology*, 73, 1103

Dane, D. S., Cameron, C. H. and Briggs, M. (1970). Virus like particles in the serum of patients with Australia antigen associated hepatitis. *Lancet*, 1, 695

Gerin, J. L., Holland, P. V. and Purcell, R. H. (1971). Australia antigen: large-scale purification from human serum and biochemical studies of its proteins. *J. Virol.*, 7, 569

Giles, J. P., McCollum, R. W., Berndtson, L. W. and Krugman, S. (1969). Viral hepatitis. Relationship of Australia/SH antigen to Willow-brook MS₂ strain. *N. Engl. J. Med.*, 281, 119

Gocke, D. J. and Kavey, N. B. (1969). Hepatitis antigen. Correlation with disease and infectivity of blood-donors. *Lancet*, 1, 1055

Hoofnagle, J. H., Gerety, R. J. and Barker, L. F. (1973). Antibody to hepatitis B virus core in man. *Lancet*, 2, 869

Hirschman, S. Z., Gerber, M. and Garfinkel, E. (1974a). DNA purified from naked intra nuclear particles of human liver infected with hepatitis B virus. *Nature*, 251, 540

Hirschman, S. Z., Vernace, S. and Schaffner, F. (1974b). DNA polymerase in preparations containing Australia antigen. *Lancet*, 1, 1099

Hirschman, S. Z. (1975). Integrator enzyme hypothesis for replication of hepatitis B virus. *Lancet*, 2, 436

Ishimaru, Y., Ishimaru, H. and Toda, G. (1976). An epidemic of infantile papular acro-dermatitis (Gianotti's disease) in Japan associated with hepatitis B surface antigen sub-type ayw. *Lancet*, **1**, 707

Kaplan, P. M., Greenman, R. L., Gerin, J. L., Purcell, R. H. and Robinson, W. S. (1973). DNA polymerase associated with human hepatitis B antigen. *J. Virol.*, **12**, 995

Krugman, S., Giles, J. P. and Hammond, J. (1967). Infectious hepatitis. Evidence for two distinctive clinical, epidemological and immunological types of infection. *JAMA*, **200**, 365

Krugman, S., Hoofnagle, J. H., Gerety, R. J., Kaplan, P. M. and Gerin, J. L. (1974). Viral hepatitis type B: DNA polymerase activity and antibody to hepatitis B core antigen. *N. Engl. J. Med.*, **290**, 1331

Le Bouvier, G. (1972). Sero analysis by immunodiffusion: the subtypes of type B hepatitis virus. In G. N. Vyas, H. A. Perkins and R. Schmid (eds.). *Hepatitis and Blood Trans-fusion*. pp 97–109. (New York: Grune and Stratton)

Le Bouvier, G. L. (1973). Subtypes of hepatitis B antigen: clinical relevance? *Ann. Intern. Med.*, **79**, 894

Magnius, L. O. and Espmark, J. A. (1972). New specificities in Australia antigen positive sera distinct from Le Bouvier determinants. *J. Immunol.*, **109**, 1017

Nielsen, J. O., Dietrichson, O. and Juhl, E. (1974). Incidence and meaning of 'e' determinant among hepatitis B antigen positive patients with acute and chronic liver diseases. *Lancet*, **2**, 913

Overby, L. R., Hung, P. P., Mao, J. C-H. and Ling, C. M. (1975). Rolling circular DNA associated with Dane particles in hepatitis B virus. *Nature*, **255**, 84

Prince, A. M. (1968). An antigen detected in the blood during the incubation period of serum hepatitis. *Proc. Natl. Acad. Sci. USA*, **60**, 814

Rizzetto, M., Canese, M. G., Arico, S., Crivelli, O., Trepo, C., Bonino, F. and Verme, G. (1977). Immunofluorescence detection of new antigen–antibody system (δ/antiδ) associated to hepatitis B virus in liver and serum of HBsAg carriers. *Gut*, **18**, 997

Robinson, W. S. and Greenman, R. L. (1974). DNA polymerase in the core of the human hepatitis B virus candidate. *J. Virol.*, **13**, 1231

PART I
Demonstration of hepatitis B virus antigens in human liver diseases

1
Methods of demonstration of hepatitis B virus components

TISSUE COLLECTION AND PROCESSING

The liver is thought to be the primary site of viral replication and synthesis: therefore hepatitis B virus antigens have been extensively sought in this organ. Among the extrahepatic organs, the antigens have been demonstrated in glomerular capillaries, the walls of blood vessels and in various lymphoid tissues. A single biopsy taken by a modified vim–silverman needle (Rake *et al.*, 1969) can be used for different immunohistochemical techniques

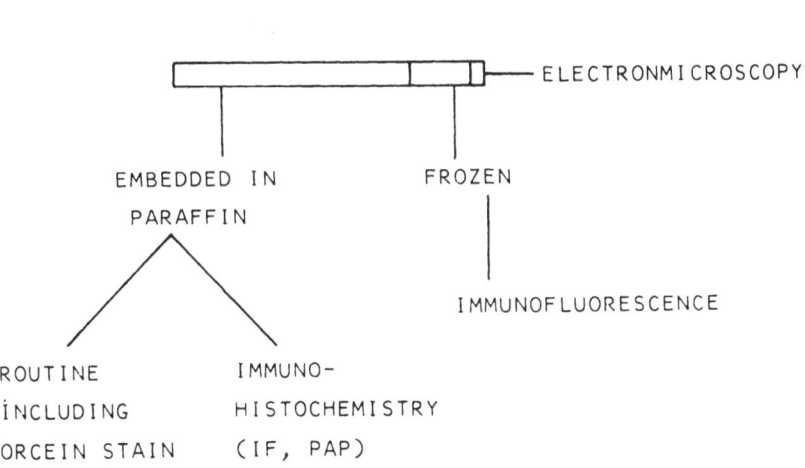

Figure 1.1 Schematic representation of a liver needle biopsy illustrating its various uses for the demonstration of HBV antigens

11

and for routine histological diagnosis. This is shown diagrammatically in Figure 1.1. For immunofluorescence the fresh specimen is frozen in iso-pentane precooled in liquid nitrogen and stored at −70°C until used. Paraffin section can also be used for immunohistochemistry and orcein stain.

ESSENTIAL IMMUNOCHEMICALS AND REAGENTS

Anti-HBs (antibody to hepatitis B surface antigen)

High titre anti-HBs obtained either from human or animal source is fairly good for the demonstration of HBsAg in tissue sections. However the specific antiserum should be checked for other tissue antibodies such as antinuclear factors, anticytoplasmic antibody and antibody against hepatitis B core antigen. An ideal antiserum should contain antibodies to both d and y subtypes.

It has found that, among the many antisera tested, anti-HBs of rabbit origin (Behringwerke) gives a strong reaction in immunofluorescence and immunoperoxidase techniques. This antiserum is used in conjunction with conjugated antirabbit globulin, e.g. goat antirabbit 7s globulin (GAR/FITC, Hyland).

Anti-HBc/FITC (antibody to hepatitis B core antigen conjugated with fluorescein)

Unlike anti-HBs, anti-HBc is not yet available commercially and is difficult to prepare in laboratory animals. The best source of anti-HBc is an acute hepatitis B convalescent patient who has just cleared the circulating HBsAg and not yet developed anti-HBs. High titre anti-HBc can also be obtained from patients with chronic aggressive hepatitis. However, in that case, to avoid infectivity, HBsAg should be separated out by ultracentrifugation. The 7s globulin fraction is extracted by an ammonium sulphate precipitation and conjugated with fluorochromes by the usual technique. As has been mentioned for anti-HBs, anti-HBc should be checked for its authenticity. Ideally the antiserum should give predominantly nuclear fluorescence in an electron microscopically proven core-positive liver.

Anti-HBs + anti-HBc

This antiserum containing antibodies against both antigens is rather difficult to procure. It is used to estimate the relative proportions of HBsAg and HBcAg present in a biopsy section. With this antiserum it is also possible to demonstrate both the antigens in a single hepatocyte. This antiserum can be used directly after conjugation with markers or indirectly in conjunction with antihuman IgG/FITC, e.g. rabbit antihuman IgG/FITC (RAHu/IgG/FITC). Application of this double antiserum yields both cytoplasmic

12

and nuclear fluorescence. Absorption either with purified HBcAg or HBsAg should abolish partially or completely the corresponding nuclear or cytoplasmic fluorescence. In the indirect method, RAHu/IgG/FITC will also detect nuclear IgG directly. This can be confirmed by incubating a serial section with RAHu/IgG/FITC alone.

Anti-immunoglobulin antisera

Both conjugated and unconjugated antiserum against individual immunoglobulins such as IgG, IgA and IgM can be obtained commercially. However, their monospecificity should be checked preferably on lymphnode biopsies of serologically proven monoclonal myelomas and lymphomas and on the basis of complete inhibition of reaction after absorption with their respective but not with different immunoglobulins.

SOLUTION FOR MODIFIED ORCEIN STAIN

Potassium permanganate solution

Potassium permanganate:	$1 \cdot 5$ g
Sulphuric acid:	$1 \cdot 5$ ml
Distilled water:	100 ml

Orcein solution

Orcein (BDH):	1 g
70% alcohol:	100 ml
Conc. HCl:	2 ml
pH $= 1-2$	

FLUORESCENCE MICROSCOPE

A good fluorescence microscope is as important as the various 'ingredients' in order to achieve a perfect immunofluorescence technique. The best combination may be found in an epi-illumination system devised by Ploem (1971), with a 6.3 × eyepiece and fitted with a HBO 200 mercury and/or XBO 75 lamp; the latter is approximately six times stronger than the former.

PROCEDURES OF DETECTION OF HEPATITIS B VIRUS COMPONENTS IN TISSUES AND BLOOD, AND CLASSIFICATION OF HEPATITIS

Hepatitis B surface antigen (HBsAg)

Immunohistochemistry–The immunohistochemical procedures include the application of immunofluorescence on both frozen and paraffin sections and immunoperoxidase on paraffin embedded liver specimens.

Immunofluorescence on frozen sections:

Conventional technique: The indirect fluorescence method was employed for the localization of HBsAg (Hadziyannis *et al.*, 1972) in the liver tissue. Sections of $4\mu m$ thickness were cut from the frozen specimen in a cryostat at $-20\,°C$, dried and processed unfixed. After washing in phosphate buffer saline (PBS) for 15 min (3 times 5 min), the slides were divided into two groups. The first group was processed by the conventional technique and the second group was used in a modified method.

For the conventional method the sections were incubated with specific anti-HBs for 45 min in a humid chamber at 30 °C, washed as above and reacted again with the appropriate FITC-conjugated antiglobulin antiserum for 30 min at room temperature. Sections were mounted in PBS–glycerine mixture after washing as before.

Modified method (Heating test): The second group of slides was put in a Coplin jar containing PBS and heated at 56°C for 30 min in a water bath. After a brief washing (to cool the slides) in PBS, incubation with FITC antiserum was performed as for the conventional method.

Specific and antiglobulin sera: Anti-HBs sera were obtained from goat, rabbit and chimpanzee. These specific antisera were used along with their respective appropriate FITC-conjugated animal antiglobulins or antihuman IgG (in the case of chimpanzee anti-HBs).

Controls and examination: Several control slides were included for specificity tests:
  (i) Incubation with normal human or normal rabbit serum instead of anti-HBs.
  (ii) Incubation with anti-HBs previously absorbed with either purified HBsAg, HBsAg positive sera or normal human serum.
  (iii) Application of FITC-conjugated heterologous antiglobulin instead of species-specific antiglobulin antisera.

Immunofluorescence on paraffin specimens:

Paraffin sections were prepared, deparaffinized and processed as for indirect immunofluorescence. The procedures and the application of different controls were the same as reported for the conventional immunofluorescence technique. In the case of paraffin sections, only rabbit anti-HBs was used.

Immunoperoxidases on paraffin sections:

The peroxidase–antiperoxidase (PAP) technique employed was basically the same as that reported by Burns (1975) and Busachi *et al.* (1978).

PAP procedure:

(i) After deparaffinization, the sections were treated with 0.5% solution of hydrogen peroxide in methanol for 15 min to block the endogenous peroxidase activity.

(ii) Background staining was diminished by applying normal swine serum for 10 min.

(iii) Sections were incubated with rabbit anti-HBs for 45 min at 30 °C.

(iv) Incubated with swine antirabbit IgG (SWAR/IgG) for 30 min at room temperature.

(v) Treated with PAP for 30 min at room temperature.

(vi) Allowed to react with diaminobenzidine for 7 min in PBS sucrose buffer.

(vii) The sections were osmicated for 10–15 s with 1% OsO_4 in phosphate buffer.

(viii) Dehydrated in graded alcohol solutions, cleared and mounted in DPX.

PBS was used for washing the sections after each incubation step.

Electronmicroscopy–Small blocks of fresh liver specimens were put immediately in 2.5% cold phosphate buffered glutaraldehyde (pH 7.2) and post fixed in 1% osmium tetroxide followed by dehydration in graded alcohols and were then embedded in epon. Ultrathin sections were cut with an ultramicrotome using diamond knives. The sections were stained with uranyl acetate (5% in distilled water) followed by lead citrate (0.3%) and examined in a Zeiss EM 10 electron microscope.

HBsAg staining with special histological dyes– Each liver biopsy processed for routine histological staining was also stained by Shikata's modified orcein stain (Shikata *et al.*, 1974).

The sections were deparaffinized and then oxided with potassium permanganate solution for 5 min. After decolourization in 2% oxalic acid, the sections were placed in orcein (BDH) solution for 4 h. The slides were dehydrated in absolute alcohol, cleared with toluene and mounted with DPX.

Demonstration of HBsAg by routine histological stains–Among the routine diagnostic stains hematoxylin–eosin (H & E) was found to allow identification of some HBsAg-containing liver cells. Such cells show a characteristic finely granular and light eosinophilic cytoplasm described as 'ground glass hepatocytes' (Hadziyannis *et al.*, 1973). The detailed morphology, frequency and diagnostic significance of this feature will be described in the next chapter.

Hepatitis B core antigen (HBcAg)

Immunofluorescence–Both direct and indirect immunofluorescence methods were applied for the demonstration of HBcAg in the frozen liver specimens. It was demonstrated by the conventional immunofluorescence technique.

Electron microscopy–HBcAg was studied by applying the same procedure as described previously for the study of HBsAg.

Demonstration of HBcAg by routine histological stains–Like 'ground glass' hepatocytes which indicate the presence of HBsAg, HBcAg-containing nuclei can also be visualized in H & E section. Such nuclei show a finely granular pale nuclear matrix termed 'sanded nuclei' by Bianchi and Gudat (1976). Unlike various nuclear inclusions, sanded material is non-membrane bound and seems to compress the chromatin against the nuclear membrane. Sanded nuclei are reported to be more frequently observed in the liver of immunosuppressed renal transplant patients than in patients with chronic hepatitis B.

Quantitation of HBsAg and HBcAg

The positive cells obtained for HBsAg as well as for HBcAg were estimated visually and expressed in approximate percentages as compared with negative cells.

Detection of HBV markers in blood

A detailed account of the various techniques applied for the demonstration of serum HBV components is not within the scope of this monograph: they are mentioned only briefly.

HBsAg

A variety of methods has been developed for the detection of HBsAg in blood. Some of the widely used tests are mentioned below:

Gel diffusion–The discovery of hepatitis B antigen (Australia antigen) was made with this test (Blumberg, 1964). Gel diffusion is simpler and cheaper than any other technique but it is time-consuming and the least sensitive.

Immunoelectrophoresis–This technique is 4–10 times more sensitive than gel diffusion. The sensitivity of the modified 'discontinuous' system is higher than the conventional method. This requires using a buffer of lower ionic strength in the supporting medium, e.g. gel, than in the tank (Combridge and Shaw, 1971). The test can be read in three hours thereby permitting its wide use especially in blood transfusion centres.

Complement fixation–The microtitre complement fixation test has been found to be more sensitive than the above mentioned methods. This test gives a quantitative measurement of the antigen in the serum allowing assessment of the course of the patient's illness.

Passive haemagglutination inhibition test–The indirect test is used for the detection of the antigen in the blood. It requires inhibition of agglutination by test sera (containing HBsAg) due to neutralization of the known antibody preparations. The test is simple and can be read in three hours.

Radioimmunoassay (RIA)–This is the most sensitive technique available for estimating circulating HBsAg. It is found to be 128 to 512 times more sensitive than gel diffusion and immunoelectrophoresis (Miller and Mordecai, 1972). The most widely used commercial radioimmunoassays are based on the solid phase technique, e.g. Austria II Abbott. This requires incubation of the test serum with anti-HBs coated plastic beads. After washing, the beads are further incubated with ^{125}I-labelled anti-HBs. The measured radioactivity is compared with a negative control. The RIA test is expensive which prevents its use in every interested laboratory.

Enzyme immunoassay–In this system, instead of a radioactive compound, an enzyme such as peroxidase or alkaline phosphatase is used to label specific anti-HBs. The test is in its experimental stage. Early data show that the sensitivity is fairly comparable to RIA (Wolters et al., 1976).

Anti-HBs

All the above methods mentioned for the estimation of HBsAg can be adjusted for the detection of anti-HBs. The passive haemagglutination method (Vyas and Shulman, 1970) and the solid phase radioimmunoassay (Ausab–Abbott) are the most widely used.

Anti-HBc

The essential step for the detection of anti-HBc in the serum is to extract HBcAg either from circulating Dane particles or from liver. The extracted purified antigen can be used to run several tests such as complement fixation, immunoelectrophoresis and radioimmunoassay (Purcell et al., 1973/74; Desmyter and Bradburne, 1975). Serum anti-HBc can also be estimated by an indirect immunofluorescence technique (Madalinsk et al., 1976).

Classification of hepatitis

Dependent upon hepatic histology, the patients were classified as cases of acute or chronic hepatitis. Each main group was further subdivided into different subgroups on the basis of previously-described morphological variations within the main groups (De Groote *et al.*, 1968; Bianchi *et al.*, 1971). Table 1.1 summarizes the classification and terminology of hepatitis used in this book.

Chronic hepatitis without cirrhosis was subdivided into chronic persistent hepatitis mainly characterized by portal inflammation and chronic aggressive hepatitis with periportal inflammation (piecemeal necrosis). Cirrhosis was classified as cirrhosis with little activity when the degree of inflammation was histologically comparable to chronic persistent hepatitis and active cirrhosis when the histology displayed piecemeal necrosis as in chronic aggressive hepatitis.

Again on the basis of predominance and proportions of hepatocellular necrosis mainly in the centrilobular area and portal tract infiltration by mononuclear cells, acute hepatitis was subdivided into three categories (Bianchi *et al.*, 1971): fully developed stage of acute hepatitis, later stage of acute hepatitis, and residual stage of acute hepatitis.

The last group – acute hepatitis with signs of possible transition to chronicity (Bianchi *et al.*, 1971; Desmet, 1973; Review, 1977) – is a histological entity combining lobular features of acute hepatitis together with periportal piecemeal necrosis.

Biopsies with minimal histological changes but numerous ground glass hepatocytes were designated as 'near normal liver'.

Table 1.1 Histological classification of chronic and acute hepatitis (De Groote *et al.*, 1968; Bianchi *et al.*, 1971)

1. CHRONIC HEPATITIS
   i. Chronic persistent hepatitis (CPH)
   ii. Chronic aggressive hepatitis (CAH)
        type A: moderate activity
        type B: severe activity
   iii. Less active cirrhosis
   iv. Active cirrhosis

1. ACUTE HEPATITIS
   i. Fully developed acute hepatitis
   ii. Later stage of acute hepatitis
   iii. Residual stage of acute hepatitis

3. ACUTE HEPATITIS WITH SIGNS OF POSSIBLE TRANSITION
   TO CHRONOCITY (AHTC)

References

Bianchi, L., De Groote, J., Desmet, V. J., Gedigk, P., Korb, G., Popper, H., Poulsen, H., Scheuer, P. J., Schmid, M., Thaler, H. and Wepler, W. (1971). Morphological criteria in viral hepatitis. Review by an international group. *Lancet*, **1**, 333

Bianchi, L. and Gudat, F. (1976). Sanded nuclei in hepatitis B. *Lab. Invest.*, **35**, 1

Blumberg, B. S. (1964). Polymorphism of serum proteins and the development of iso-precipitins in transfused patients. *Bull. N.Y. Acad. Med.*, **40**, 377

Burns, J. (1975). Background staining and sensitivity of the unlabelled antibody sandwich method using formalin fixed paraffin embedded material. *Histochemistry*, **43**, 291

Busachi, C. A., Ray, M. B. and Desmet, V. J. (1978). An immunoperoxidase technique for demonstrating membrane localized HBsAg in paraffin section of liver biopsies. *J. Immunol. Met.*, **19**, 95

Combridge, B. S. and Shaw, C. (1971). Immunoelectro-osmophoresis using discontinuous buffer system to detect Australia antigen in pooled human plasma. *Lancet*, **2**, 1189

De Groote, J., Desmet, V. J., Gedigk, P., Korb, G., Popper, H., Poulsen, H., Scheuer, P. J., Schmid, M., Thaler, H., Wehlinger, T. and Wepler, W. (1968). A classification of chronic hepatitis. *Lancet*, **2**, 626

Desmet, V. (1973). Chronic hepatitis (including primary biliary cirrhosis). In E. A. Gall and F. K. Mostofi (ed.). *The Liver*. (Baltimore: Williams and Wilkins)

Desmyter, J. and Bradburne, A. F. (1975). Core antibodies and other parameters of hepatitis B virus infection in a tropical population. *Develop. Biol. Standard*, **30**, 194

Hadziyannis, S., Vissoulis, C. H., Moussouros, A. and Afroudakis, A. (1972). Cytoplasmic localization of Australia antigen in the liver. *Lancet*, **1**, 976

Hadziyannis, S., Gerber, M. A., Vissoulis, C. and Popper, H. (1973). Cytoplasmic hepatitis B antigen in ground glass hepatocytes of carriers. *Arch. Path.*, **96**, 327

Madalinski, K., Budkowska, A., Michaelak, K. T. and Trepo, C. (1976). Immunofluorescent test for the detection of anti-HBc in HBs antigen subtypes. *Biblio. Haemat.*, **42**, 57

Miller, J. P. and Mordecai, B. G. (1972). Evaluation of a solid phase radioimmunoassay technique for the detection of hepatitis associated antigen. *J. Nucl. Med.*, **13**, 454

Ploem, J. S. (1971). A study of filters and light sources in immunofluorescence microscopy. *Ann. N.Y. Acad. Sci.*, **77**, 414

Purcell, R. H., Gerin, J. L., Almeida, J. B. and Holland, P. V. (1973/74). Radio-immunoassay for the detection of core of the Dane particle and antibody to it. *Inter-virology*, **2**, 231

Rake, M. O., Murray-Lyon, I. M., Ansell, I. D. and Williams, R. (1969). Improved liver biopsy needle. *Lancet*, **2**, 1283

Review by an International Group (1977). Acute and chronic hepatitis revisited. *Lancet*, **2**, 914

Shikata, T., Uzawa, T., Yoshiwara, N., Akatsuka, T. and Yamazaki, S. (1974). Staining method of Australia antigen in paraffin section. Detection of cytoplasmic inclusion bodies. *Jap. J. Exp. Med.*, **44**, 25

Vyas, G. N. and Shulman, N. K. (1970). Haemagglutination assay for antigen and antibody associated with viral hepatitis. *Science*, **170**, 332

Wolters, G., Kunpers, L. and Schuurs, A. (1976). Solid-phase enzyme immunoassay for detection of hepatitis B surface antigen. *J. Clin. Path.*, **29**, 873

2
Evaluation of the various procedures for the demonstration of hepatitis B surface antigen and hepatitis B core antigen in liver tissue

DEMONSTRATION OF HEPATITIS B SURFACE ANTIGEN

Immunofluorescence

Immunofluorescence on frozen sections

There exists a proven link between HBsAg and serum hepatitis or hepatitis B. However, contact with HBV produces diverse reactions in the host (Dudley *et al.*, 1971; Hoofnagle *et al.*, 1975). HBsAg may remain undetectable in the serum even by as sensitive a technique as radioimmunoassay in a significant number of patients with clinical hepatitis even when longitudinal studies and the evolution of HB antibodies suggests HBV as the causative agent (Hoofnagle *et al.*, 1975). Sometimes HBsAg could not be detected in the liver of hepatitis B patients despite the presence of the antigen in the body fluids (Krawczynski *et al.*, 1972). On the contrary the absence of the antigen in the serum does not exclude its presence in the liver (Ray *et al.*, 1976a; Ray *et al.*, 1976b). Although these discrepancies in the findings may be due to varying degrees of interactions between the host immune system and the virus (Blumberg *et al.*, 1970; Dudley *et al.*, 1971), serum HBsAg may be masked by components of normal serum proteins such as complement factors (Miller *et al.*, 1972) and certainly by anti-HBs itself (Shorey and Combes, 1973) and thus may

21

remain undetectable by immunological methods. This study was undertaken to improve the demonstration of HBsAg in liver tissue and was achieved by adding a tissue heating step to the conventional fluorescence antibody technique.

Materials and methods–Biopsy selection and processing: 84 frozen liver biopsies were included in this study.

Results

Conventional method: HBsAg localization: of 84 biopsies, 40 (48%) were positive. HBsAg was demonstrable in variable amounts in the cytoplasm and at the cell membrane of the hepatocytes. Sometimes fluorescence was restricted to the perinuclear zone or only at the sinusoidal pole of the liver cells. The intensity of the fluorescence varied from biopsy to biopsy. No specific fluorescence was demonstrated in the nuclei of the liver cells by using antisera of animal origin. The incidence of positive reactions and the relation between the various distribution patterns of HBsAg with different histological types of hepatitis will be described in Chapter 3.

Table 2.1   Summary of the results obtained by the conventional and the modified fluorescence test

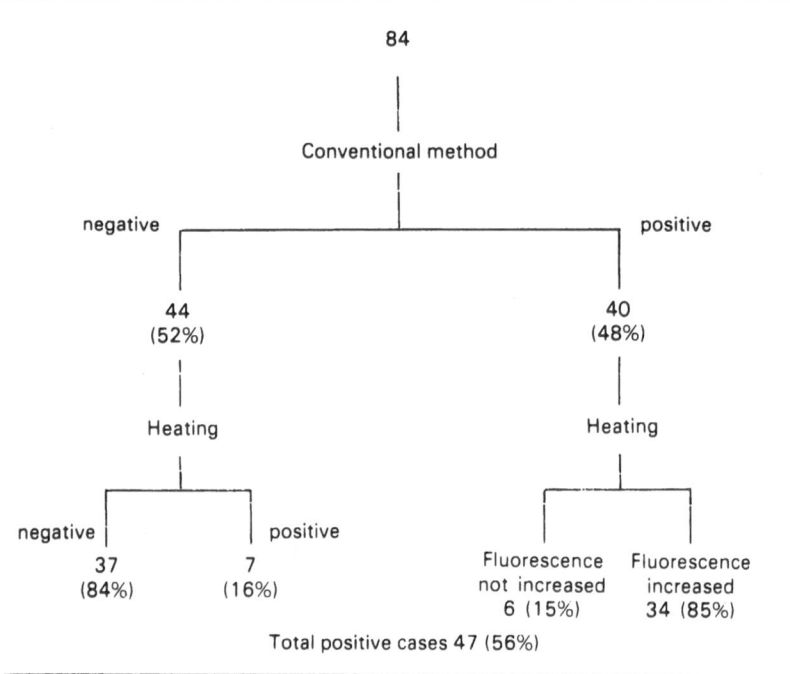

Effect of heating (modified method): Table 2.1 summarizes the results obtained both by the conventional method and after heating. In 85% (34 of 40) the intensity of the fluorescence was increased after heating and the number of positive cells was increased as well (Figures 2.1a, 2.1b). Some doubtful cases became frankly positive. The background non-specific fluorescence diminished considerably. No increase in the intensity of fluorescence or in the number of positive cells was obtained in 15% (6 cases) of the positive biopsies. Of 44 biopsies negative by the conventional method, 16% (7 cases) became positive after heating (Figures 2.2a, 2.2b).

Specificity of fluorescence: The fluorescence was considered specific for HBsAg when it was either partially or completely abolished after absorption of specific antisera with HBsAg positive sera. No fluorescence was observed when specific antisera were replaced by either normal human sera or normal rabbit serum. The same was found when inappropriate conjugated antiglobulins were used instead of antiglobulins of appropriate specificity.

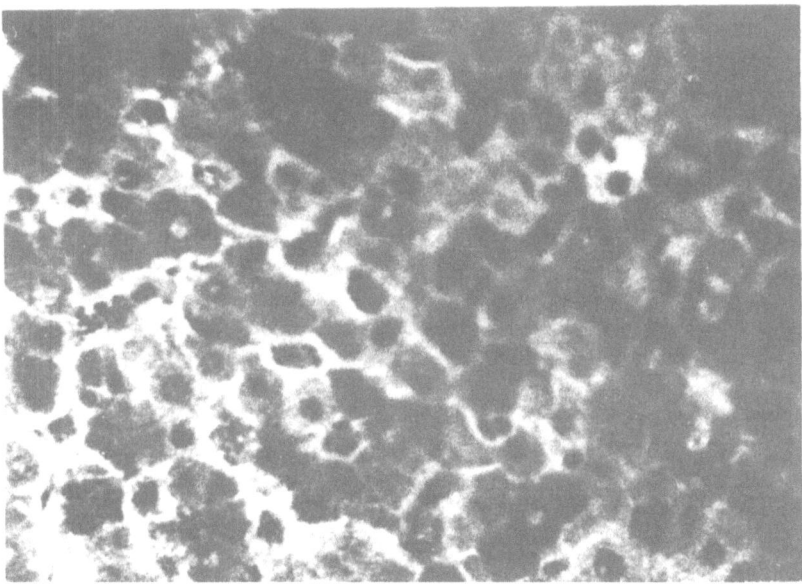

Figure 2.1a Conventional fluorescence method: HBsAg specific granular fluorescence is present in the cytoplasm. Intense reaction is observed in the cell membrane (× 570)

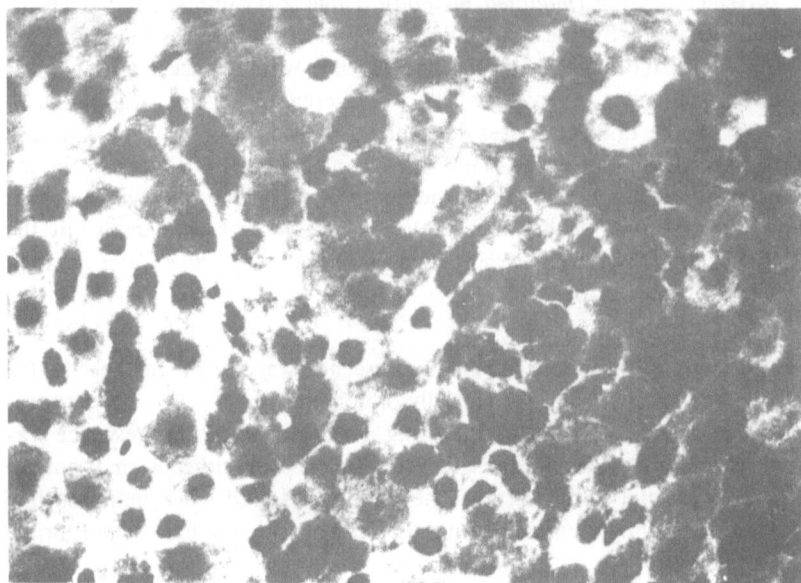

Figure 2.1b Serial section of the same biopsy as in Figure 2.1a, after heating shows bright cytoplasmic fluorescence with clearly defined cell outlines and diminished background compared to Figure 2.1a (×570)

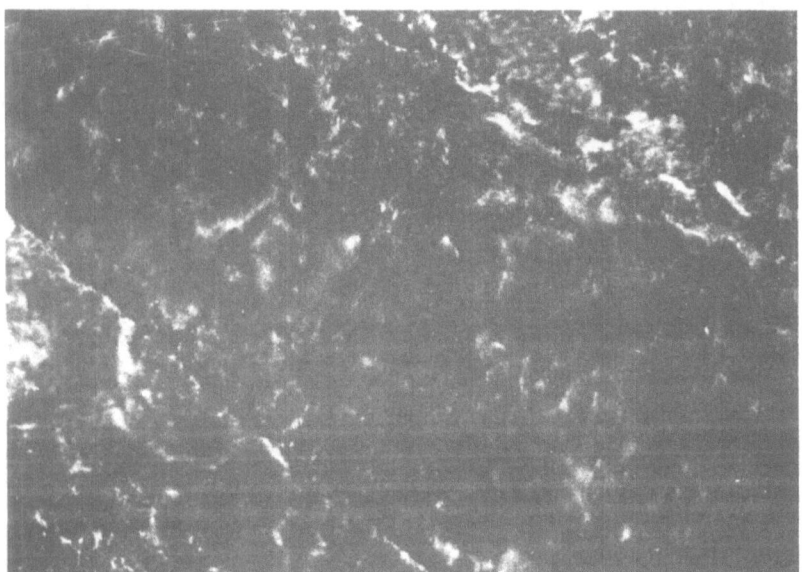

Figure 2.2a Conventional method : no specific fluorescence for HBsAg is detected in the hepatocytes (×570)

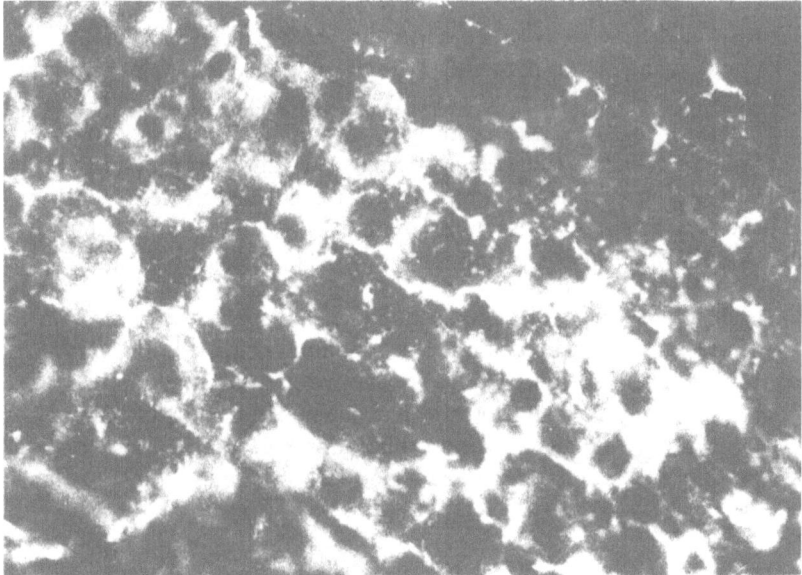

Figure 2.2b Serial section of the same biopsy as in Figure 2.2a after heating shows bright cytoplasmic fluorescence in the hepatocytes (×570)

Discussion—The results obtained indicate that the modified method is more sensitive than the usual fluorescence technique. With the conventional as well as with the modified procedures, HBsAg was localized in the cytoplasm and the cell membrane of the hepatocytes. The application of the pre-heating step increased the intensity and crispness of the fluorescence and some biopsies, negative by the conventional method, became clearly positive after heating.

Several authors have reported masked HBsAg in the serum which escapes detection by ordinary immunological methods (Miller *et al.*, 1972; Ziegenfuss, 1972). Various factors, including complement, have been incriminated in this masking effect. Shorey and Combes (1973) have postulated that anti-HBs itself can cover up the antigen in the serum. Heating produced additional positives in the present study, but the mechanisms of the unmasking of the antigen in the hepatocytes is not known at present. It is possible that destruction or elimination of complement occurs at the site of antigen–antibody reaction (Nowoslawski *et al.*, 1972) after heating; alternatively, some other tissue factor may mask the antigen. It may be that the heating makes more antigenic sites available to react effectively.

Immunofluorescence on paraffin sections

HBsAg was detected in sera stored for 25 years (Zuckerman and Taylor, 1969) and found to be resistant to many physical and chemical agents (Kim and Bissel, 1971). It is destroyed by heating only at 80–100 °C. (Zuckerman, 1972). Therefore it was thought that the antigenicity of HBsAg might remain unaltered through the entire process of paraffin embedding after routine fixation and still remain detectable by immuno-histochemical procedures. Paraffin sections would be preferable for their easy manipulation and better preservation of histological details.

Materials and methods–Biopsy selection and examination: 20 liver biopsies, 10 positive and 10 negative for HBsAg by immunofluorescence on frozen sections, were investigated. Both the positive and negative biopsies were collected in the same period of time and the maximum age of the paraffin blocks used was one year. Orcein staining for HBsAg in paraffin sections was performed according to Shikata and co-workers (1974).

Results

HBsAg in frozen sections: The intrahepatic localization patterns of HBsAg are described above under the heading conventional and modified immunofluorescence techniques.

HBsAg in paraffin sections: The 10 biopsies previously shown to contain HBsAg in frozen sections were also positive in paraffin sections even in cases where the fluorescence on frozen sections was rather weak. The HBsAg-containing hepatocytes had a similar distribution pattern (Figures 2.3 and 2.4a). However, the intensity of the fluorescence, especially for the membrane-localized HBsAg, appeared slightly weaker than in frozen sections. The histological localization of the fluorescent cells was easier and more precise. Non-specific fluorescence was negligible and the control reactions were negative. Ten biopsies, previously found to be HBsAg negative in frozen sections, were also negative in paraffin sections.

HBsAg localization by orcein staining: The demonstration of HBsAg by orcein staining will be reported in detail in the next section dealing with the localization of HBsAg with histological dyes. The results are mentioned here to make a comparison with the immunofluorescence findings. The results obtained by immunofluorescence and orcein staining are summarized in Table 2.2. Of the 10 biopsies which were positive in both frozen and paraffin sections, only six were positive by orcein staining. The orcein positive cells in serial sections (Figures 2.4a, 2.4b). Smaller amounts of antigen, especially in the liver cell membrane, detected by immunofluorescence (Figure 2.5) did not stain with orcein,

26

which only showed intensely positive cells. However, with orcein stain the exact histological location of the positive cells was easy to determine.

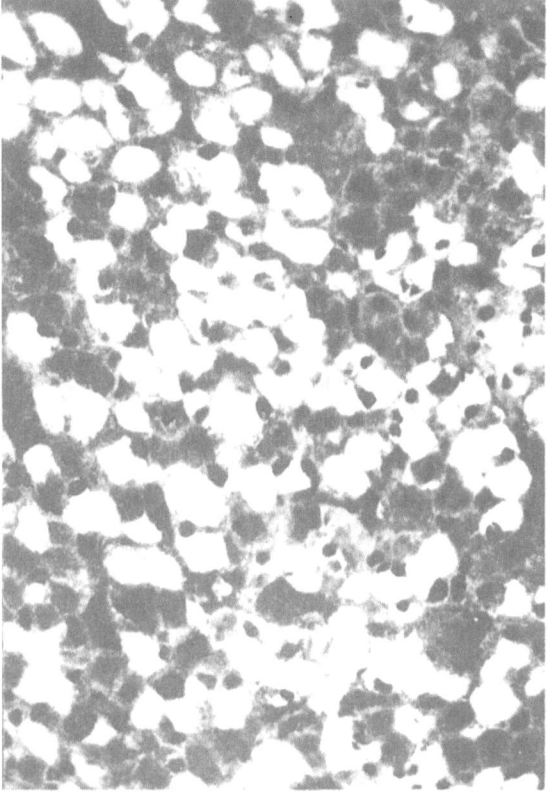

Figure 2.3 Frozen section : HBsAg specific fluorescence is strong and homogeneous in character and occupies variable portions of the cytoplasm (×230)

Discussion–This study reports an immunofluorescence technique for the demonstration of HBsAg in paraffin-embedded liver tissue, fixed in the widely-used Bouin's solution. The results obtained are identical to those obtained in frozen sections, except for a slight decrease in the intensity of the reaction. The immunofluorescent test on paraffin sections has several practical advantages:

(i) Paraffin sections are easily cut with an ordinary microtome and freezing equipment is not necessary.

(ii) The precise location of the antigen is easily delineated as there is only slight shrinkage of the paraffin-embedded tissue.

27

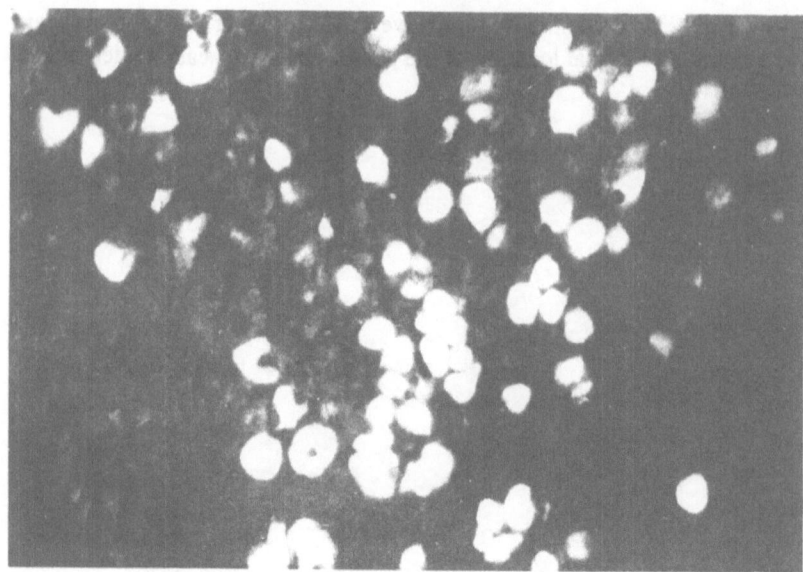

Figure 2.4a Paraffin section of the same biopsy as in Figure 2.3. Processed 10 months after collection, shows a similar pattern of fluorescence in the cytoplasm (× 230)

Table 2.2 Summary of the results for HBsAg obtained by immunofluorescence in frozen sections and by immunofluorescence and orcein staining in paraffin sections

| | | Paraffin sections | | | |
| | | Immunofluorescence | | Orcein | |
Frozen sections	Number	Positive	Negative	Positive	Negative
Immunofluorescence positive	10	10	0	6	4
Immunofluorescence negative	10	0	10	0	10
TOTAL	20				

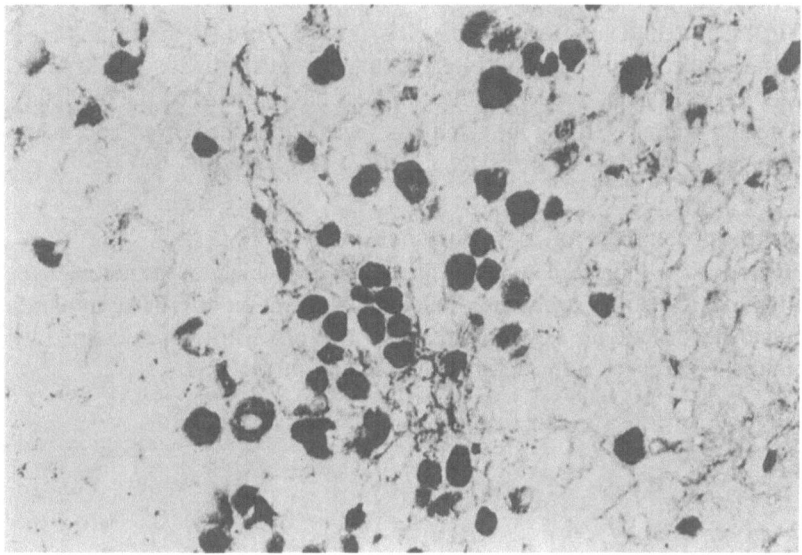

Figure 2.4b Orcein staining: serial section from the same biopsy cylinder as in Figure 2.4a, shows dark brown globules in the cytoplasm of the hepatocytes. These cells correspond to the fluorescent hepatocytes in Figure 2.4a (× 230)

(iii) Preservation of histological detail is better than in frozen section.

(iv) Referred biopsies sent by mail can be examined by immunofluorescence.

(v) Paraffin blocks at least one year old retain positivity. However, subsequent investigation has shown that HBsAg could be demonstrated in liver specimens stored for 20 years at room temperature.

(vi) There is less danger of spread of infection than with frozen sections of fresh, unfixed tissues from hepatitis patients. Hence, numerous complicating precautions are unnecessary when paraffin sections are used.

(vii) The use of serial paraffin sections allows an easier comparative study of routine H & E slides and slides stained for HBsAg. Nevertheless, some membrane staining may be missed after using paraffin sections.

Admittedly, the advantages enumerated above may also be valid for the orcein method (Shikata *et al.*, 1974). However, the immunofluorescence technique applied in this study has the unquestionable advantage of immunological specificity. Moreover, from these results it also appears to have a clearly higher sensitivity. Finally it should be stressed that the paraffin sections used in this study were taken from routinely processed tissues without any special manoeuvres such as have been prescribed by Sainte-Marie (1962).

After our present original report, others (Huang, 1975; Huang *et al.*, 1976) reported demonstration of HBsAg and HBcAg in formol-fixed, paraffin-embedded specimens after treatment with pronase and trypsin. In the course of time, several other workers have confirmed the feasibility of demonstrating HBsAg in fixed and wax embedded liver specimens (Portmann *et al.*, 1976; Buffet *et al.*, 1977; Molas *et al.*, 1977).

Immunoperoxidase on paraffin sections

This study was undertaken to investigate the applicability of the peroxidase–antiperoxidase (PAP) procedure for the demonstration of HBsAg in paraffin-embedded material and to compare the results with those obtained by immunofluorescence both in frozen and paraffin sections.

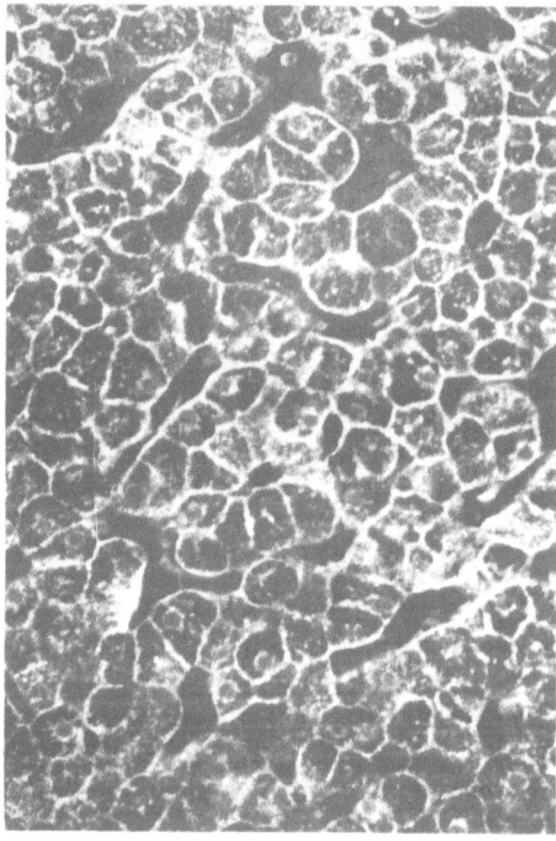

Figure 2.5 Paraffin section : processed one year after collection. Shows membrane-localized HBsAg in the hepatocytes (× 230)

Materials and methods–Fifteen liver specimens in which HBsAg was previously localized in the cytoplasm and liver cell membranes in frozen sections by the modified immunofluorescence technique were selected for this investigation. The biopsies were histologically diagnosed as chronic aggressive hepatitis (9 cases) and active cirrhosis (6 cases).

Twenty other biopsies of miscellaneous liver disorders (chronic aggressive hepatitis, active cirrhosis, alcoholic liver disease, hepatocellular carcinoma) but negative for HBsAg both in the liver and blood, served as controls.

Results–In the PAP method, specific positivity was observed as dark brown deposits at the site of DAB reaction (Figure 2.6). Osmication enhanced the intensity of the histochemical reaction, allowing a clear identification of the positive cells. Both cytoplasmic and membrane-localized HBsAg were visualized. The results obtained by immunofluorescence and PAP techniques are summarized in Table 2.3. Of the 15 biopsies in which both cytoplasmic and membrane-localized HBsAg were previously demonstrated 'on frozen sections', all were positive in the cytoplasm by both techniques. However membrane-localized HBsAg was demonstrable only in 7 by immunofluorescence and in 8 by the PAP method. All immunofluorescent positive specimens were also positive in PAP.

The control reactions and all the control biopsies were negative. Occasionally erythrocytes and Kupffer cells showed faintly positive peroxidase reactions.

Discussion–The results obtained in the present study confirm the observation by Burns (1975), Afroudakis *et al.* (1976) and Busachi and co-workers (1978) on the suitability of the PAP technique for the demonstration of HBsAg in fixed material. The data further show that the application of the immunofluorescence method in paraffin section is as sensitive as the PAP procedure. With reference to the demonstration of membrane-localized HBsAg, both the techniques described above are found to be less sensitive than immunofluorescence performed on frozen unfixed specimens. Although the PAP method requires a few more steps than the usual immunofluorescent procedure, its application is simple and the slides can be examined in an ordinary light microscope. The greatest advantage of this technique is that a permanent preparation can be obtained.

The intracellular localization patterns of HBsAg obtained in the present investigation by the PAP method are similar to previous observations (Burns, 1975; Afroudakis *et al.*, 1976; Busachi *et al.*, 1978), in which was reported strong cytoplasmic positivity with faint membranous reaction. However in contrast to these findings two recent studies (Tapp and Jones, 1977; Blenkinsopp and Hoffenden, 1977) have failed to demonstrate membrane-localized HBsAg by both indirect immunoperoxidase and PAP techniques in formol fixed paraffin embedded material.

Table 2.3 Comparison of results obtained in paraffin sections by immunofluorescence and PAP techniques

Diagnosis	No. of biopsies	Frozen sections	Paraffin sections			
		Immunofluorescence	Immunofluorescence		PAP	
		Membrane + Cytoplasm	Cytoplasm	Membrane	Cytoplasm	Membrane
Hepatitis	15	15	15	7	15	8
Miscellaneous	20	—	—	—	—	—

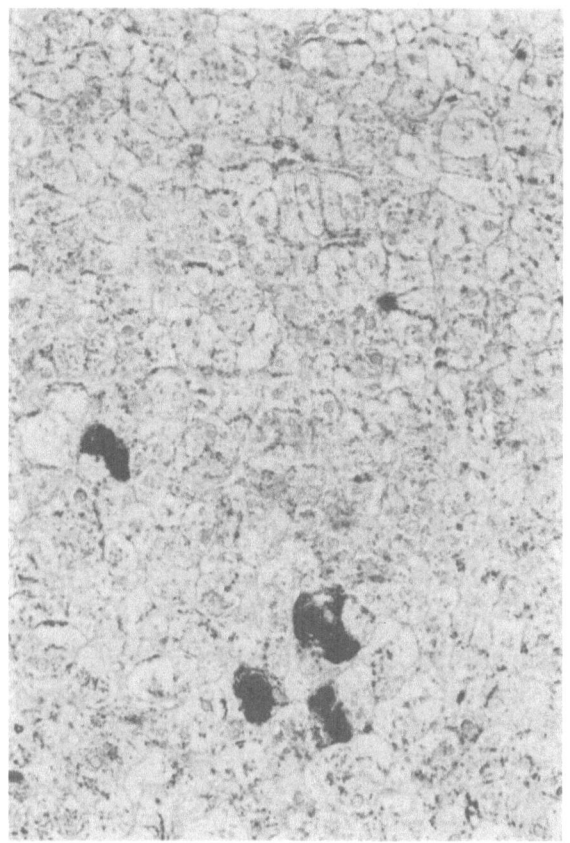

Figure 2.6 Paraffin section: PAP method: dark brown staining specific for HBsAg is present in the liver cell membrane. Few hepatocytes show cytoplasmic positivity (× 230)

Demonstration of HBsAg with special histological dyes (orcein stain)

Until 1974, HBsAg was localized in tissue sections by relatively complicated procedures requiring immunohistochemistry and electron microscopy. However, the introduction of several histological stains by Shikata and co-workers (1974) has greatly simplified the techniques for demonstrating HBsAg in conventional paraffin sections. Table 2.4 shows the various histological methods employed for the demonstration of HBsAg in ordinary paraffin embedded material. All these staining procedures, in particular the modified orcein stain (Shikata *et al.,* 1974), can be performed in any histology laboratory. This part deals with the efficacy and drawbacks of

33

the orcein stain in comparison with other immunohistochemical procedures applied on paraffin section.

Materials—A total of 150 orcein positive liver biopsies collected from various histological types of hepatitis were reviewed for the present investigation.

Results—HBsAg-containing hepatocytes stained dark brown and corresponded to the fluorescent cells in the serial section (Figures 2.4a, 2.4b), confirming the specificity of the orcein stain. The distribution patterns of HBsAg observed by orcein staining were similar to those seen by immunofluorescence. The amount and the intensity of orcein positivity varied from biopsy to biopsy, and even from area to area in the same biopsy. Typical

Table 2.4 Different staining procedures applied for the demonstration of HBsAg in paraffin sections (Shikata *et al.*, 1974)

1. Orcein stain

2. Aldehyde–fuchsin method

3. Aldehyde–thionine method

4. Alcian B blue method

5. Resorcin–fuchsin method

membrane-localized HBsAg, which was frequently observed in chronic aggressive forms of hepatitis B by immunohistochemical techniques, was not observed after orcein staining. In agreement with immunofluorescent results, a higher amount (both at cellular and lobular levels) of HBsAg was found in less active forms than in active forms of hepatitis B; orcein positivity was not observed in the liver of patients with acute hepatitis B.

The location of the positive cells was more precise and more clearly visible in the orcein sections than in immunofluorescence. In histologically 'near normal liver' with a large number of ground glass hepatocytes and in some cases of CPH, it was possible to formulate a rough idea of the lobular topography of the orcein positive cells. They were frequently observed around the central vein especially in zones 3 and 2 of the liver acinus of Rappaport (Figure 2.7). However, as on immunofluorescence, this phenomenon was not observed in CAH and active cirrhosis which were usually characterized by a low amount of HBsAg and a random, spotty distribution of positive cells. The relative sensitivity of the orcein stain compared to immunofluorescence in fixed material was described in the previous Section of this Chapter (Table 2.2). It has been observed that orcein stained only cells containing a high amount of HBsAg, present in aggregated forms as in ground glass hepatocytes, whereas a small amount of antigen dispersed throughout the hepatocytic cytoplasm especially in cases with active cirrhosis was not detectable with orcein.

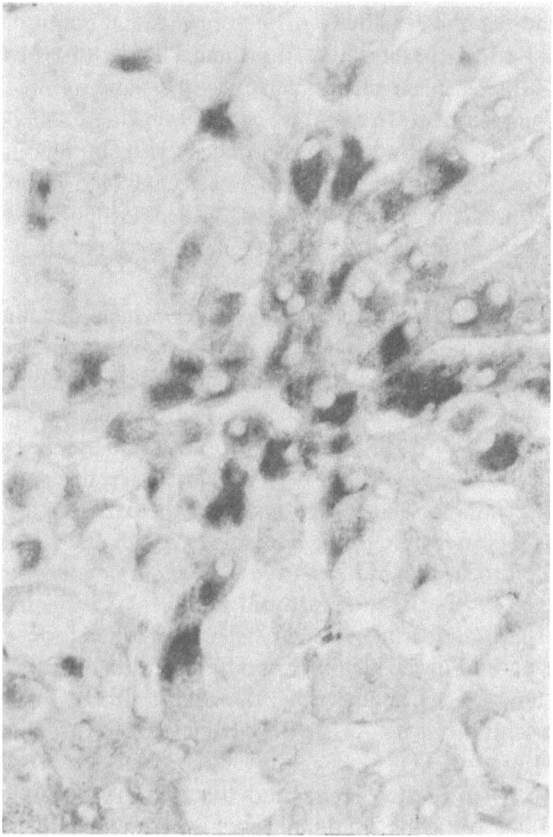

Figure 2.7 Orcein staining : orcein positivity specific for HBsAg is present in the hepatocytes in zones 3 and 2 of the liver acinus of Rappaport (× 230)

Non-specific background staining varied from biopsy to biopsy. Sometimes macrophages and hepatocytes containing bile pigment or lipofuscin gave intense staining, resulting in false positive reactions. Elastic tissue present both in the central vein and portal tracts stained strongly.

Discussion—The staining of the same cell both by orcein and by immunofluorescence confirms the affinity of the dye for HBsAg. The exact mechanism of staining of HBsAg containing hepatocytes by orcein is unknown. Shikata and co-workers (1974) suggested the involvement of disulphide bonds.

Indeed, HBsAg has been shown to contain high levels of the amino acid cystine which contains disulphide bonds (Dreesman *et al.*, 1972; Vyas *et al.*, 1972). Orcein also has an affinity for other structures rich in disulphide bonds such as keratin of hair follicles and elastic fibres.

Regarding the relative sensitivity of the orcein stain, contradictory data have been reported in the literature. Portmann *et al.*, (1976) found that the number of HBsAg positive specimens was the same by orcein staining as by immunofluorescence. On the other hand, Nayak and Sachdeva (1975) observed a higher positivity with orcein than with immunofluorescence or immunoperoxidase. Our findings and two recent reports on the application of the orcein stain (Buffet *et al.*, 1977; Blenkinsopp and Hoffenden, 1977) immunohistochemical methods are more sensitive than the orcein stain.

The orcein stain has many practical values which include all those mentioned in the previous section dealing with the advantages of performing immunohistochemistry on fixed tissue. Recently, orcein staining has been found to have diagnostic value. On the basis of the paucity of HBsAg in the liver of patients with acute hepatitis B and its abundance in chronic hepatitis and the carrier state, it has been suggested that this simple method is useful in differentiating acute hepatitis from the carrier state (Deodhar *et al.*, 1975) and acute from chronic hepatitis (Kostich and Ingham, 1977). Furthermore the orcein dye has been found to stain copper–protein complexes (Sipponen, 1976) present mostly in the liver of patients with long-standing cholestasis and primary biliary cirrhosis. Therefore, it has been considered to be useful in the histological differentiation of extra- and intra-hepatic cholestasis and primary biliary cirrhosis from orcein-negative, non-cholestatic chronic liver diseases including CAH (Salaspuro and Sipponen, 1976).

In conclusion, it must be emphasized that the greatest advantage of the orcein method over the immunohistochemical techniques lies in its simplicity which makes is suitable for use in any routine histology laboratory.

Demonstration of HBsAg by routine histological stains

A 'ground glass' appearance of the liver cells has been found to be associated with the presence of excess amounts of HBsAg (Hadziyannis *et al.*, 1973) in the cytoplasm. These cells can easily be identified in sections stained routinely with H & E. This part deals with the morphology, occurrence and diagnostic significance of the ground glass hepatocytes found in the liver of various types of hepatitis B.

Morphology

The characteristic appearance of the ground glass hepatocytes has been reviewed recently by Thomsen *et al.* (1976). In the light microscope the positive cells show a uniform, finely granular light eosiniophilic cytoplasm contrasting with the bluish cytoplasm of the surrounding normal liver cells (Figure 2.8). In most cases, only a part of the cytoplasm is affected and often a clear space separates the glassy area from the cell periphery. The ground glass areas correspond to the fluorescent and orcein positive cells. The nucleus remains unaffected and is occasionally situated eccentrically.

Ground glass hepatocytes are also stainable with Gomori's aldehyde fuchsin (Shikata *et al.*, 1974) and aldehyde thionine (Winckler *et al.*, 1976).

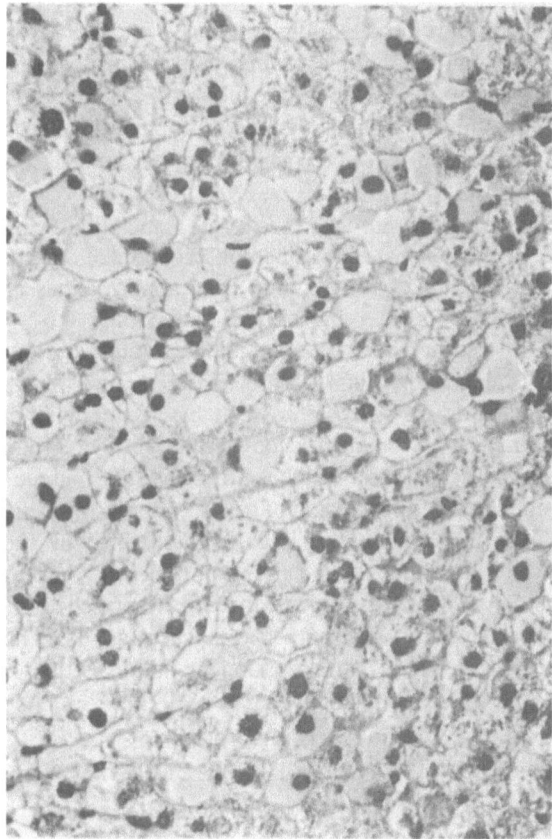

Figure 2.8 HBsAg containing 'ground glass hepatocytes'. The positive cells show a uniform granular. light eosinophilic cytoplasm: H & E (× 230)

Distribution patterns

The distribution patterns of ground glass hepatocytes vary from biopsy to biopsy, even from area to area in the same biopsy. In most cases, the cells occur in clusters with predominant localization in zone 2 of the liver acinus of Rappaport. Larger numbers of ground glass cells are observed in 'near normal liver' obtained from healthy HBsAg carriers, and moderate numbers in CAH; they are absent in acute hepatitis B. The incidence of ground glass hepatocytes in relation to hepatocellular necrosis will be described in Chapter 4.

Discussion

The existence of ground glass hepatocytes was first noticed by Klinge and Bannasch (1968) in the liver of individuals who had received large doses of drugs such as barbiturates, sulphonamides and corticosteroids which were known to stimulate the microsomal biotransformation system and to induce proliferation of the smooth endoplasmic reticulum (SER). Subsequently such 'induced' cells were reported in patients undergoing therapy with the chlorpromazin (Popper, 1973) and rifampicin (Scheuer et al., 1974).

The discovery of ground glass cells in association with the HBsAg carrier state is indeed rewarding since observation of such cells in otherwise healthy individuals with minimal liver abnormalities is sufficient to assume the presence of intercurrent HBV infection.

The 'induced' cell and HBsAg-containing ground glass hepatocytes are histologically similar. They can only be differentiated by the presence or absence of reactions for HBsAg as seen by immunohistochemistry and orcein staining. In electron microscopy both types of ground glass cells show pronounced hyperplasia of the smooth endoplasmic reticulum, reduction of mitochondria and repression of rough endoplasmic reticulum. Nevertheless, the HBsAg-containing cells can be identified by the presence of typical intracisternal filaments and round particles (Thomsen et al., 1976).

In conclusion, although the significance of the presence of ground glass hepatocytes depends on different factors such as positive or negative reaction for HBsAg, their demonstration in tissue section is useful as a diagnostic hint for HBV infection (Popper, 1975).

DEMONSTRATION OF HEPATITIS B CORE ANTIGEN

Immunofluorescence

HBcAg was detected in the liver of HBsAg positive patients both by immunofluorescence and by electron microscopy. With immunofluorescence,

HBcAg was detected mostly in the nuclei of the hepatocytes and rarely in the cytoplasm and membrane of the liver cells. The nuclear fluorescence was granular and of variable intensity (Figure 2.9). In most instances no fluorescence was observed in the nucleoli and occasionally full nuclear positivity was obtained. The positive nuclei were distributed in groups or appeared scattered throughout the liver lobules. There seemed to be no correlation between the distribution of the positive nuclei and a particular lobular topography (centrilobular or periportal area).

HBcAg specific fluorescence was also observed in the cytoplasm of the hepatocytes as bright green fluorescent granules (Figure 2.10) arranged in groups or scattered all over the hepatocytic cytoplasm. The majority of hepatocytes showing positive cytoplasmic staining were also positive

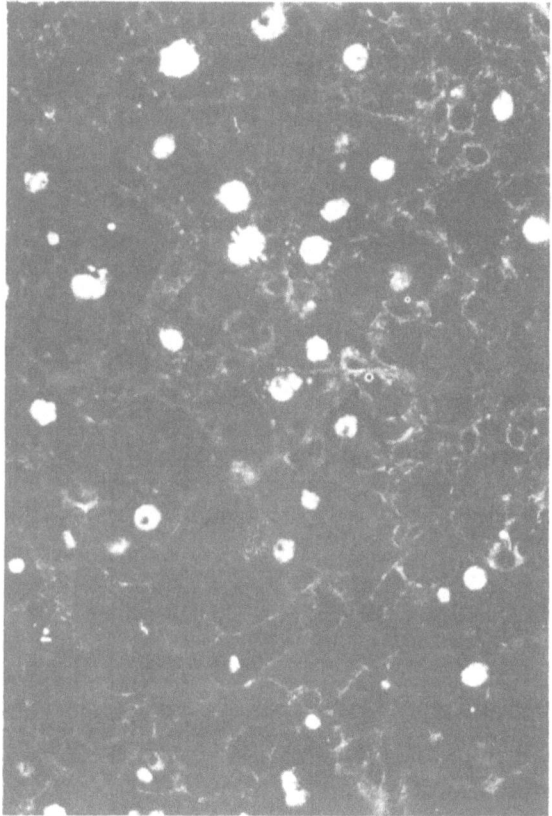

Figure 2.9 Liver biopsy from a patient with CAH treated with immunosuppressive agents. HBcAg specific fluorescence of variable intensity limited to the nuclei of the hepatocytes. Nucleoli remain dark (× 230)

for the nucleus and in only a few was the cytoplasm alone positive. HBcAg fluorescence was also observed in the periphery of the hepatocytes as tiny beads arranged in chains, and even in the sinusoidal space.

Simultaneous demonstration of HBcAg and HBsAg

By applying anti-HBc and anti-HBs, it was possible to localize both HBcAg and HBsAg in the same hepatocytes. In this procedure, the specific fluorescence was green in colour for both antigens. However, when contrast colour fluorochromes were used, HBsAg and HBcAg appeared red and green respectively (this will be discussed in detail in Chapter 5). With double stainings, most of the hepatocytes showed single staining: either

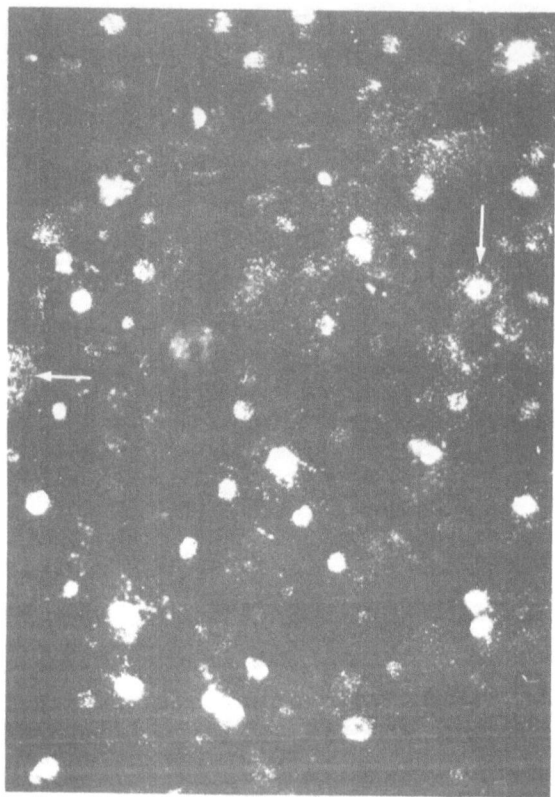

Figure 2.10 Liver biopsy from a patient with active cirrhosis treated with immunosuppressive drugs. HBcAg is visualized both in the nuclei and in the cytoplasm of some hepatocytes. Cytoplasmic HBcAg is granular and unevenly distributed all over the cytoplasm and is observed even in the periphery of the hepatocytes (arrows) (× 230)

40

for nuclear HBcAg or for cytoplasmic HBsAg. Only very few cells gave a specific reaction for both HBcAg and cytoplasmic HBsAg (Figure 2.11). However, when membrane-localized HBsAg was taken into account, then the number of such doubly stained cells was found to be relatively high.

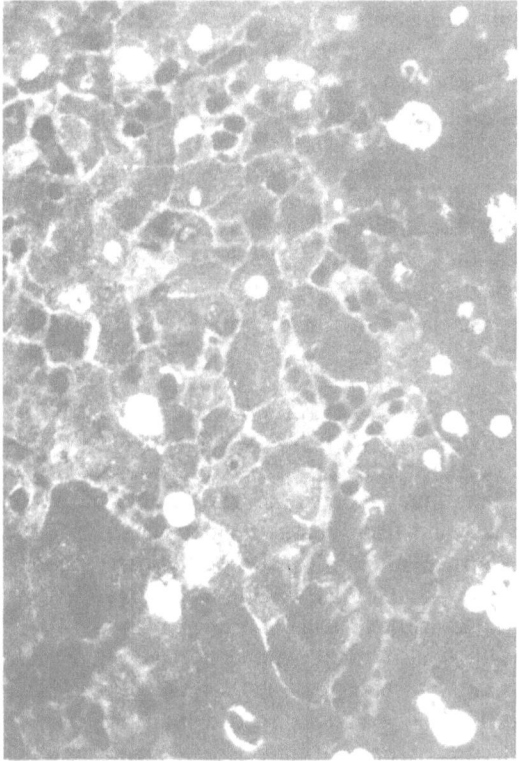

Figure 2.11 Biopsy from a patient with active cirrhosis treated with immunosuppressive drugs. Both HBsAg and HBcAg are observed in the same hepatocytes. HBsAg is present also on the liver cell membrane (× 230)

Demonstration of HBcAg and HBsAg by regular electron microscopy

Immunohistochemical (Ray and Desmet, 1975; Ray *et al.*, 1976c) and histological procedures (Shikata *et al.*, 1974; Deodhar *et al.*, 1975) have been most commonly employed to demonstrate HBV antigens in liver specimens. These studies detected HBsAg in the cytoplasm and membranes of the hepatocytes and HBcAg in the nuclei and rarely in the cytoplasm of the liver cells (Ray *et al.*, 1976c). However, light microscopic techniques are inadequate to visualize individual cell organelles involved in the synthesis and transport of viral antigens. Therefore both regular (Huang *et al.*, 1974; Gudat *et al.*, 1975) and immune electron microscopic investigations (Gerber *et al.*, 1974) have been applied in the past.

The present electron microscopic study (De Vos *et al.*, 1979) was undertaken on biopsies positive by immunofluorescence in order to investigate the exact ultrastructural location of the viral components in the hepatocytes and to obtain some insight in the site of synthesis of both HBsAg and HBcAg, their assembly and ultimate transport as complete virus into the circulation.

Materials and methods—Fifteen liver biopsies, in which HBsAg was demonstrated in the cytoplasm as well as in the cell membranes and HBcAg in the nuclei and/or cytoplasm by immunofluorescence on frozen sections, were selected for this investigation.

Results

Demonstration of HBcAg: in each liver biopsy a varying number of hepatocytes contain particles of 21–25 nm in size, mostly in the nuclei. As observed in immunofluorescence, the number of such particles varies from cell to cell and from biopsy to biopsy. Most of the particles are empty, some of them are full. These particles correspond to the core particles described by Gudat *et al.* (1975). Occasionally, a few core particles are demonstrated in the nuclear pores (Figure 2.12). These uncoated core particles are also found in the hyaloplasm even up to the cell periphery at the sinusoidal pole and in the pericanalicular ectoplasm. A few core particles could also be demonstrated in the canalicular lumen. Most core particles lying in the hyaloplasm are non-coated or naked.

However, a few of the core particles appeared to be surrounded by a narrow rim of semidense material. Such particles are occasionally observed in the perinuclear hyaloplasm but mostly localized in the cell periphery near the sinusoidal space and in the intercellular space and Disse's space. No naked cores are visible inside the endoplasmic vesicles or perinuclear space.

Still another type of core particle apparently covered by a well defined outer membrane is visualized in the hepatocytic cytoplasm. They are few in number and invariably observed inside the vesicles of the endoplasmic reticulum mostly situated at the periphery of the cell. They resemble Dane particles seen in the sera.

42

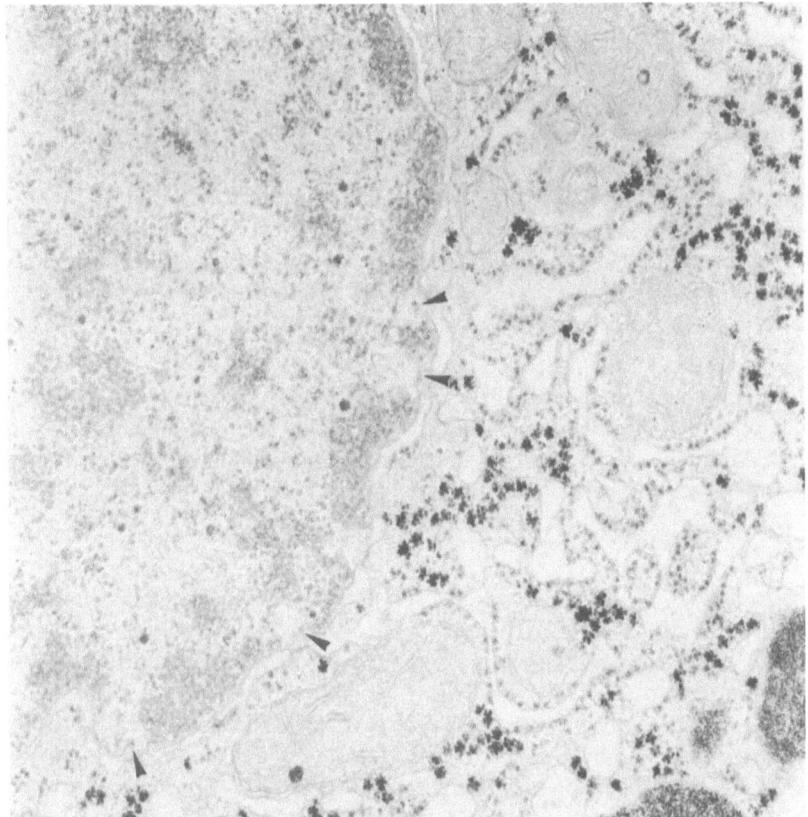

Figure 2.12 Biopsy from a patient with CAH: ultrastructural demonstration of non-coated core particles in the hepatocytic nucleus. Such particles are also observed in the nuclear pores; indicated by arrows (× 36 400)

Demonstration of HBsAg: In 8 of the 15 biopsies longitudinally cut tubules and cross section of HBsAg are found in the cisternae of the SER. The number of these particles varied from cell to cell and even from area to area in a single hepatocyte (Figure 2.13). True filaments and the cross-sectional forms characteristic of HBsAg are not observed in the periphery of the cell. However, in most of the hepatocytes the peripheral cytoplasm beneath the cell membrane thickened, apparently by the deposition of disorganized microfilamentous material. In some areas, variable amounts of amorphous material could be seen in a widely dilated intracellular space. No structural forms of HBsAg are observed outside the cell. Thickening of the membrane with hypertrophic filamentous material could also be found to a lesser extent in cells without

43

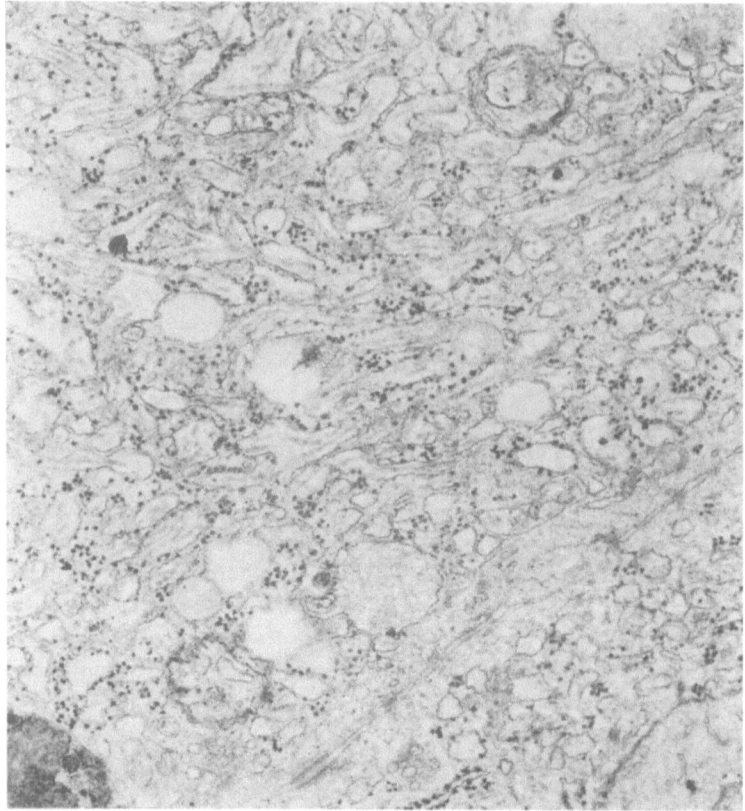

Figure 2.13 Biopsy from a patient with less active cirrhosis : HBsAg characteristic intra-cisternal filaments and encapsulated forms, which may be the cross section of the filaments, are present within the SER (× 36 400)

typical HBsAg tubules in the cytoplasm proper. Filamentous or cross sectional forms are never obscured in the hepatocytic nuclei.

Discussion–The electron microscopic study demonstrates characteristic filaments and round particles, probably representing longitudinal and cross sections of the HBsAg filaments in the cytoplasm, and HBcAg particles mostly in the nuclei and occasionally in the cytoplasm of the liver cell. These filamentous structures and core particles have been found to be immunologically identical to HBsAg and HBcAg respectively (Gerber et al., 1974; Barker et al., 1974). The localization of HBsAg and HBcAg at the ultrastructural level corroborates the findings obtained by immuno-fluorescence study (Gudat et al., 1975; Ray et al., 1976c).

The exact sites of synthesis of HBV antigens are not well understood. However, based on their usual preferential location, it is believed that HBcAg (core particles) is synthesized in the hepatocytic nucleus and HBsAg (filaments) in the cytoplasm (Hirschman, 1975). In the present study abundant core particles are observed in the nucleus, rarely in the nuclear pores and moderately but clearly in the cell cytoplasm and cell periphery. The cytoplasmic naked core particles are always demonstrated in the hyaloplasm but not inside the endoplasmic reticulum profiles.

These findings may indicate that HBcAg is synthesized in the nucleus and transported through the cytoplasm towards the cell surface and ultimately released into the circulation by some unknown mechanism. This contention is substantiated by the observation of core particles outside the cell in the intercellular and Disse's spaces and in the sinusoidal space. However, such free naked core particles were not observed by electron microscopic examination of serum rich in Dane particles (Hirschman et al., 1974).

On the other hand the presence of core particles in the hyaloplasm and in the nuclear pores may also suggest that HBcAg is synthesized in the cytoplasm and subsequently migrates into the nucleus for maturation, travels back to the cytoplasm and is released into the blood. This phenomenon has recently been observed for herpes simplex (Tooze, 1973) and SV_{40} (Tabuchi et al., 1976) in which the viral proteins are synthesized on free polysomes and membrane-bound ribosomes and then migrate into the nucleus.

In a recent immunoelectron microscopic examination performed with peroxidase-labelled anti-HBc, Yamada and Nakane (1977) have observed non-structural forms of HBcAg in the ribosomes and formulated the same hypothesis.

In this investigation core particles surrounded by electron dense material resembling Dane particles were seen inside the cisternae of the endoplasmic reticulum. These large particles are frequently present in the vicinity of the cell periphery. This finding may suggest that the 42 nm Dane particle is probably formed at the periphery of the cell.

HBsAg is represented by the filaments present both in the hepatocytes and in the circulation. The presence of HBsAg specific filaments inside the SER suggests that this viral component is probably synthesized as small units, assembled into long tubules and ultimately transported into the circulation. However, true structural forms of HBsAg are not visualized at the cell periphery although considerable amounts of membrane-localized HBsAg are observed in the cell membrane by immunofluorescence.

In conclusion electron microscopic investigation has confirmed the previously described (Ray et al., 1976c) immunofluorescence findings. It allows a more precise localization of HBV components in the intracellular compartments. However, the dynamics of HBV synthesis, intracellular transport and elimination into the circulation require further elucidation.

References

Afroudakis, A. P., Choong-Tsek Liew, P. S. and Peters, R. L. (1976). An immunoperoxidase technic for the demonstration of the hepatitis B surface antigen in human livers. *Am. J. Clin. Path.*, **65**, 533

Barker, L. F., Almeida, J. D., Hoofnagle, J. H., Gerety, R. J., Jackson, R. and McGrath, P. P. (1974). Hepatitis B core antigen : immunology and electronmicroscopy. *J. Virol.*, **14**, 1552

Blenkinsopp, W. K. and Hoffenden, G. P. (1977). Aetiology of cirrhosis, hepatic fibrosis and hepatocellular carcinoma. *J. Clin. Path.*, **30**, 579

Blumberg, B. S., Sutnick, A. I. and London, W. T. (1970). Australia antigen as a hepatitis virus. Variation in host response. *Am. J. Med.*, **48**, 1

Buffet, C., Briantais, M. J., Chaput, J. C., Rain, B., Martin, E. and Etienne, J. P. (1977). Détection des antigénes HBs et HBc dans des biopsies hépatiques humaines par immunofluorescence et coloration par l'orcéine. *Gastroenterol. Clin. Biol.*, **1**, 127

Burns, J. (1975). Immunoperoxidase localisation of hepatitis B antigen in formalin paraffin processed liver tissue. *Histochemistry*, **44**, 133

Busachi, C. A., Ray, M. B. and Desmet, V. (1978). An immunoperoxidase technique for demonstrating membrane localized HBsAg in paraffin section of liver biopsies. *J. Imm. Met.*, **19**, 95

Deodhar, K. P., Tapp, E. and Scheuer, P. J. (1975). Orcein staining of hepatitis B antigen in paraffin sections of liver biopsies. *J. Clin. Path.*, **29**, 66

De Vos, R., Ray, M. B. and Desmet, V. J. (1979). Electron microscopy of hepatitis B virus components in chronic active liver disease. *J. Clin. Path.*, (in press)

Dreesman, G. R., Hollinger, B., Surinao, J. R., Fujjoka, R. S. Brunschwig, J. R. and Melnick, J. L. (1972). Biophysical and biochemical heterogeneity of purified hepatitis B antigen. *J. Virol.*, **10**, 469

Dudley, F. J., Fox, R. A. and Sherlock, S. (1971). : Relationship of hepatitis-associated antigen (HAA) to acute and chronic liver injury. *Lancet.*, **2**, 1

Gerber, M. A., Hadziyannis, S., Vissoulis, C., Schaffner, F., Paronetto, F. and Popper, H. (1974). Electron microscopy and immune electron microscopy of cytoplasmic hepatitis B antigen in hepatocytes. *Am. J. Path.*, **75**, 489

Gudat, F., Bianchi, L., Sonnabend, W., Thiel, G., Aenishaenslin, W. and Stalder, G. A. (1975). Pattern of core and surface expression in liver tissue reflects state of specific immune response in hepatitis B. *Lab. Invest.*, **32**, 1

Hadziyannis, S., Gerber, M. A., Vissoulis, C. and Popper, H. (1973). Cytoplasmic hepatitis B antigen in 'ground glass' hepatocytes of carriers. *Arch. Pathol.*, **96**, 327

Hirschman, S. Z. (1975). Integrator enzyme hypothesis for replication of hepatitis B virus. *Lancet*, **2**, 436

Hirschman, S. Z., Gerber, M. and Garfinfel, E. (1974). Purification of naked intranuclear particles from human liver infected by hepatitis B virus. *Proc. Nat. Acad. Sci. USA*, **71**, 3345

Hoofnagle, J. H., Gerety, R. J. and Barker, L. F. (1975). Antibody to hepatitis B core antigen. *Am. J. Med. Sci.*, **270**, 179

Huang, S. (1975). Immunohistochemical demonstration of hepatitis B core and surface antigens in paraffin sections. *Lab. Invest.*, **33**, 88

Huang, S., Groh, V., Beaudoin, J. G., Dauphinee, W. D., Guttmann, R. B., Morehouse, D. D., Aronoff, A. and Gault, H. A. (1974). A study of the relationship of virus-like particles and Australia antigen in liver. *Hum. Path.*, **5**, 209

Huang, S. N., Minassian, H. and More, J. D. (1976). Application of immunofluorescent staining on paraffin sections improved by trypsin digestion. *Lab. Invest.*, **35**, 383

Kim, C. Y., Bissel, D. M. (1971). Stability of the lipid and protein of hepatitis-associated (Australia) antigen. *J. Infect. Dis.*, **123**, 470

Klinge, O. and Bannasch, P. (1968). *In Verhandlungen der deutschen Gesellschaft für Pathologie*, pp. 568–573. (Stuttgart: G. Fischer Verlag)

Kostich, N. and Ingham, C. D. (1977). Detection of hepatitis B surface antigen by means of orcein staining of liver. *Am. J. Clin. Path.*, **67**, 20

Krawczynski, K., Nazarewicz, T., Brzosko, W. J. and Nowoslawski, A. (1972). Cellular localization of hepatitis associated antigen in livers of patients with different forms of hepatitis. *J. Infect. Dis.*, **126**, 372

Miller, J. E., Rossman, D. P., Ziegenfuss, J. F. and Kenworthy, H. J. (1972). Serum hepatitis with 'masked' Australia antigen. *J. Am. Med. Assoc.*, **221**, 916

Molas, G., Voillemot, N. and Potet, F. (1977). Identification de l'antigène HBs par immuno-fluorescence indirecte sur coupes de foie inclus en paraffine au cours des différentes formes d'hépatite virale. *Gastroenterol. Clin. Biol.*, **1**, 249

Nayak, N. C. and Sachdeva, R. (1975). Localization of hepatitis B surface antigen in conventional paraffin sections of the liver. *Am. J. Path.*, **81**, 479

Nowoslawski, A., Krawczynski, K., Brzosko, W. J. and Madalinski, K. (1972). Tissue localization of Australia antigen immune complexes in acute and chronic hepatitis and liver cirrhosis. *Am. J. Path.*, **68**, 31

Popper, H. (1973). In E. A. Gall and F. K. Mostofi (eds.) *The Liver*. pp. 182–198. (Baltimore: Williams and Wilkins Co.)

Popper, H. (1975). The ground glass hepatocyte as a diagnostic hint. *Hum. Path.*, **6**, 517

Portmann, B., Galbraith, R. M., Eddleston, A. L. W. F., Zuckerman, A. J. and Williams, R. (1976). Detection of HBsAg in fixed liver tissue – use of a modified immunofluorescent technique and comparison with histochemical methods. *Gut*, **17**, 1

Ray, M. B. and Desmet, V. J. (1975). Immunofluorescent detection of hepatitis B antigen in paraffin-embedded liver tissue. *J. Immunol. Met.*, **6**, 283

Ray, M. B., Desmet, V. J., Fevery, J., De Groote, J., Bradburne, A. J. and Desmyter, J. (1976a). Hepatitis B surface antigen (HBsAg) in the liver of patients with hepatitis : a comparison with serological detection. *J. Clin. Path.*, **29**, 89

Ray, M. B., Desmet, V. J., Fevery, J., De Groote, J., Bradburne, A. J. and Desmyter, J. (1976b). Distribution patterns of hepatitis B surface antigen (HBsAg) in the liver of hepatitis patients. *J. Clin. Path.*, **29**, 94

Ray, M. B., Desmet, V. J., Bradburne, A. F. Desmyter, J., Fevery, J. and De Groote, J. (1976c). Differential distribution of hepatitis B surface antigen and hepatitis B core antigen in the liver of hepatitis B patients. *Gastroenterology*, **71**, 462

Sainte-Marie, G. (1962). A paraffin embedding technique for studies employing immuno-fluorescence. *J. Histochem. Cytochem.*, **10**, 250

Salaspuro, M. and Sipponen, P. (1976). Demonstration of an intracellular copper-binding protein by orcein staining in long-standing cholestatic liver diseases. *Gut*, **17**, 787

Scheuer, P. J., Lal, S., Summerfield, J. A. and Sherlock, S. (1974). Rifampicin hepatitis, clinical and histological study. *Lancet*, **1**, 421

Shikata, T., Uzawa, T., Yoshiwara, N., Akatsuka,, T. and Yamazaki, S. (1974). Staining methods of Australia antigen in paraffin sections – detection of cytoplasmic inclusion bodies. *Jap. J. Exp. Med.*, **44**, 25

Shorey, J. and Combes, B. (1973). Selective heat inactivation of hepatitis B antibody (HBAB) in sera containing both hepatitis B antigen (HBAG) and HBAB (abstract). *Hepatologie*, **1**, 238

Sipponen, P. (1976). Orcein positive hepatocellular material in long-standing biliary diseases. *Scand. J. Gastroent.*, **1**, 546

Tabuchi, K., Lehman, J. M. and Kirsch, W. M. (1976). Immunocytochemical localization of simian virus 40 T antigen with peroxidase-labelled antibody fragments. *J. Virol.*, **17**, 668

Tapp, E. and Jones, D. M. (1977). HBsAg and HBcAg in the livers of asymptomatic hepatitis B antigen carriers. *J. Clin. Path.*, **30**, 671

Thomsen, P., Poulsen, H. and Petersen, P. (1976). Different types of ground glass hepatocytes in human liver biopsies : morphology, occurrence and diagnostic significance. *Scand. J. Gastroent.*, **11**, 113

Tooze, J. (1973). *The Molecular Biology of Tumour Viruses*, pp. 481. (New York: Cold Spring Harbor Laboratory)

Vyas, G. N., Rao, K. R. and Ibrahim, A. B. (1972). Australia antigen : a conformational antigen dependent on disulphide bonds. *Science*, **178**, 1300

Winckler, K., Junge, U. and Creutzfeldt, W. (1976). Ground glass hepatocytes in unselected liver biopsies. Ultrastructure and relationship to hepatitis B surface antigen. *Scand. J. Gastroent.*, **11**, 167

Yamada, G. and Nakane, P. K. (1977). Hepatitis B core and surface antigen in liver tissue: light and electron microscopic localization by the peroxidase labeled antibody method. *Lab. Invest.*, **36**, 649

Ziegenfuss, J. F. (1972). Testing for Australia antigen. *Br. Med. J.*, **2**, 48

Zuckerman, A. J. (1972). In *Hepatitis-associated Antigen and Viruses*. p. 73. (Amsterdam: North-Holland)

Zuckerman, A. J. and Taylor, P. E. (1969). Persistence of the serum hepatitis (SH-Australia) antigen for many years. *Nature*, **223**, 81

3
Hepatitis B surface antigen in the liver and serum of patients with hepatitis

The first part of this chapter deals with the incidence of HBsAg in the blood as well as in the liver of patients with hepatitis. The second part describes the various intrahepatic patterns of expression of HBsAg in hepatitis B.

HEPATITIS B SURFACE ANTIGEN IN THE LIVER OF PATIENTS WITH HEPATITIS: A COMPARISON WITH SEROLOGICAL DETECTION

Wide variations have been found in the incidence of HBsAg in the serum of the patients with acute (Shulman and Barker, 1969; Prince *et al.*, 1970; Mossor-Ostrowska *et al.*, 1974; Wenzel *et al.*, 1975) and chronic (Sutnick *et al.*, 1969; Velasco and Katz, 1970; Wewalka *et al.*, 1970) hepatitis. The frequency of HBsAg in chronic hepatitis as estimated in the blood varies from 4% in Australia (Cooksley *et al.*, 1975) to 62% in Austria (Wewalka *et al.*, 1970). Table 3.1 summarizes the incidence of serum HBsAg in the normal population as well as in chronic hepatitis patients in different countries as determined by various serological methods.

The variation in the reported incidence of HBsAg may be due to differences in the geographical prevalence of HBV infection (Cooksley *et al.*, 1975) and/or differences in the technique used for estimation (Prince, 1971).

In the liver tissue, the antigen was consistently detected by immunofluorescence in various forms of HBsAg sero-positive chronic hepatitis (Hadziyannis *et al.*, 1972; Krawczynski *et al.*, 1972) suggesting that immunofluorescence may compete with serology in the ability to detect HBsAg in those patients. There are conflicting reports regarding the demon-

49

stration of HBsAg in the liver of acute hepatitis with circulating HBsAg (Coyne et al., 1970; Krawczynski et al., 1972; Cérat et al., 1973; Mossor-Ostrowska et al., 1974; Gudat et al., 1975). In the present study, a comparison has been made between the immunofluorescent demonstration of HBsAg in the liver of hepatitis patients and the serological detection of HBsAg by radioimmunoassay (Ling and Overby, 1972). In chronic hepatitis, an attempt has been made to correlate the HBsAg status and the histological type of the disease with sex, gammaglobulin and transaminase values and the presence of tissue antibodies.

Material and methods

Two hundred and forty-six liver biopsies obtained from patients with various hepatic dysfunctions were included in this study. The patients were mostly adults of Belgian origin.

Serology: Blood from each patient was collected within a week of performing liver biopsy. In each serum sample HBsAg was assayed by RIA. Sera from each patient were also assayed for tissue antibodies, i.e. ANF (antinuclear factor), AMA (antimitochondrial antibody) and SMA (smooth muscle antibody) by indirect immunofluorescence.

Results

Of the 246 liver biopsies examined, 100 were from patients with histologically proven acute or chronic hepatitis and the remaining 146 were from patients with a wide variety of other liver disorders. The results of HBsAg immunofluorescence in the tissue and circulating HBsAg in hepatitis patients are given in Table 3.2. Further results, e.g. transaminase gammaglobulins and auto-antibodies, on chronic hepatitis patients are given in Table 3.3. On the basis of immunofluorescence and serology, the biopsies in each subgroup of patients were divided into four categories : liver and serum positive, liver positive but serum negative, liver negative but serum positive, and liver and serum both negative. No consistent histological differences were found between HBsAg positive and HBsAg negative biopsies.

In chronic hepatitis HBsAg was detected in 52 of 76 patients (68%) by immunofluorescence and in 40 by RIA (57%). In all RIA positive cases, HBsAg could be detected with immunofluorescence; 12 of the 52 (23%) tissue positive cases could not be detected by RIA in the serum. The detection of HBsAg in the liver of patients devoid of demonstrable circulating antigen was specific as shown by various specificity tests; also HBsAg was not observed in the liver of 146 patients without hepatitis. The highest incidence of HBsAg was obtained in CAH (70%) and in active cirrhosis

(79%). A higher frequency of HBsAg in more active forms, compared to less active forms, was found in chronic hepatitis with and without cirrhosis and attained statistical significance ($p \sim 0.05$). No significant correlation was found between HBsAg status and levels of transaminases, gammaglobulins and tissue antibodies (Table 3.3). In chronic hepatitis, 51 patients were males and 25 were females: 72% of males and 60% of females were HBsAg positive.

In acute hepatitis (including AHTC), HBsAg was detected in 8 out of 24 patients (33%) with immunofluorescence and in 12 with RIA (50%). All immunofluorescence positive cases could be detected with RIA. In the fully developed stage of acute hepatitis, 4 out of 5 HBsAg positive cases could be detected only by RIA. The later stage of acute hepatitis, and AHTC, although histologically distinct, resemble chronic hepatitis in that HBsAg was detectable both in the liver and in the serum (Table 3.2).

Discussion

In chronic hepatitis as a whole, the frequency of HBsAg as obtained with immunofluorescence (68%) and RIA (57%) is comparable with the incidence reported from other parts of central and east europe (Wewalka et al., 1970; Bianchi et al., 1972). The reported results were obtained by estimating the circulating antigen with methods as sensitive as the complement fixation test and immunoelectrophoresis. Thus the differences in the sensitivity of the techniques used cannot be invoked as the only cause of variation in the frequency of HBsAg in chronic hepatitis (Reed et al., 1973; Cooksley et al., 1975). The normal frequency of HBsAg in Belgium as determined by RIA is 0.4–0.5% (unpublished data), which is comparable to figures reported from Australia (Mason et al., 1972) and USA (Ling and Overby, 1972). Therefore the high frequency of HBsAg obtained in chronic hepatitis in the population examined cannot be ascribed to a high prevalence of HBV infection in this area. The variation in the frequency may be due to differences in the genetic make-up of the patients (Reed et al., 1973) or to other unknown factors. Whatever may be the explanation, this study shows a high incidence of HBsAg in patients with chronic hepatitis.

HBsAg positive patients with chronic hepatitis have been described as both younger (Bianchi et al., 1972) and older (Sherlock et al., 1970) than HBsAg negative patients. Gammaglobulin levels have been found to be lower in HBsAg positive cases than in HBsAg negative cases (Bulkley et al., 1970) and auto-antibodies to be absent in the blood of HBsAg positive cases but present in HBsAg negative cases (Bulkley et al., 1970; Wright, 1970; Cooksley et al., 1972). Such differences were not found in the present study.

Table 3.1 Incidence of HBsAg in normal population and in chronic hepatitis in different countries

Country	Normal incidence %	Methods	Chronic hepatitis No.	Positive %	Methods	Authors
Australia	0.11	IEOP	85	4	RIA	Cooksley et al. 1975
Austria	0.46	IEOP	34	62	IEOP	Wewalka et al. (1970)
Belgium	0.5	RIA	76	57 in blood*	RIA	Ray et al. (1976a)
Great Britain	<1	RIA	94	18	RIA	Reed et al. (1973)
Italy	1.5	IEOP	59	51	IEOP	Bianchi et al. (1972)
Scandinavia	0.6	RIA	206	24	RIA	Skinhoj et al. (1977)
USA	0.3–1	RIA	30	23	CF, ID	Bulkley et al. (1970)

*68% in liver by immunofluorescence

Table 3.2 Histological diagnosis and frequency of HBsAg obtained by serology and immunofluorescence

Histological diagnosis	Numbers	Liver+ Serum+	Liver+ Serum−	Liver− Serum+	Liver+	Serum+	Both Liver Serum−
1. CHRONIC HEPATITIS							
(a) Chronic persistent hepatitis	11	4	2	—	6(55%)	4(36%)	5(45%)
(b) Chronic aggressive hepatitis	20	12	2	—	14(70%)	12(60%)	6(30%)
(c) Cirrhosis with little activity	11	3	2	—	5(45%)	3(27%)	6(55%)
(d) Active cirrhosis	34	21	6	—	27(79%)	21(62%)	7(21%)
Total	76	40	12	—	52(68%)	40(57%)	24(32%)
2. ACUTE HEPATITIS							
(a) Fully developed stage of acute hepatitis	7	1	—	4	1(14%)	5(71%)	2(29%)
(b) Later stage of acute hepatitis	9	4	—	—	4(44%)	4(44%)	5(56%)
(c) Residual stage of acute hepatitis	3	—	—	—	—	—	3(100%)
3. ACUTE HEPATITIS WITH SIGNS OF POSSIBLE TRANSITION TO CHRONICITY	5	3	—	—	3(60%)	3(60%)	2(40%)
Total	24	8	—	4	8(33%)	12(50%)	12(50%)
4. MISCELLANEOUS	146	—	—	—	—	—	146(100%)

Table 3.3 Comparison of age, sex, biochemical features and auto-antibodies in HBsAg positive (both in liver and serum) and negative chronic hepatitis

Diagnosis	IFT	Serology	Number	Age mean (range)	Sex Male	Sex Female	Gammaglobulins (g/100ml)	SGOT† (IU/l)	SGPT† (IU/l)	Auto-antibodies ANF+	AMA+	SMA+	(Nr)*
CPH	+	+	4	34(17–48)	3	1	1.58 ± 0.34	37 ± 15	69 ± 47	—	—	—	(3)
	+	–	2	54(51–57)	1	1	1.48 ± 0.52	9 ± 1	9 ± 1	—	—	—	(1)
	–	–	5	43(30–58)	4	1	1.95 ± 0.57	21 ± 14	39 ± 32	2	—	—	(4)
CAH	+	+	12	46(15–58)	7	5	1.66 ± 0.33	61 ± 44	117 ± 103	3	—	—	(7)
	+	–	2	64(61–66)	1	1	2.01 ± 0.50	19 ± 1	35 ± 9	—	—	—	(2)
	–	–	6	43(16–53)	3	3	1.84 ± 0.72	49 ± 60	81 ± 85	2	—	1	(5)
Active	+	+	3	51(33–62)	2	1	2.20 ± 0.93	27 ± 15	33 ± 18	—	—	—	(1)
Cirrhosis	+	–	2	51(37–64)	2	0	1.00 ± 0.08	17 ± 0	19** ± 2	—	—	—	(1)
	–	–	6	55(44–66)	3	3	1.16 ± 0.26	15 ± 8	13** ± 2	—	—	—	(3)
Cirrhosis with	+	+	21	53(30–70)	17	4	2.19 ± 0.95	72 ± 58	101 ± 74	1	—	—	(12)
little	+	–	6	42(22–63)	4	2	2.48 ± 1.33	76 ± 64	80 ± 71	2	1	—	(4)
activity	–	–	7	45(19–69)	4	3	1.68 ± 0.64	84 ± 145	80 ± 116	—	2	1	(4)

* Numbers in brackets denote number of cases tested for autoantibodies
** Value significantly different from the group with positive serology ($p < 0.05$)
† Normal values for SGOT and SGPT are below 19 IU/l and 24 IU/l respectively

There were no morphological differences between HBsAg positive and HBsAg negative biopsies. The highest incidence of HBsAg was seen in active cirrhosis which was the prevalent type in this series. These findings contrast apparently with those of Bianchi et al., (1972) who reported cirrhotic changes most frequently in antigen negative groups. HBsAg was more frequently present in patients with CAH or active cirrhosis than in those with CPH and less active cirrhosis. However, the amount of HBsAg in the hepatocytes was higher in less active forms (Ray et al., 1976b).

In twelve patients with chronic hepatitis HBsAg could be detected in the liver but not in the serum. These cases could not be sharply segregated from others on the basis of histological, epidemiological and biochemical parameters. In this study, the most sensitive methods available were used to estimate HBsAg in the liver and blood; yet a number of cases of chronic hepatitis remain HBsAg negative in the serum. This does not necessarily mean that HBV infection is not present in HBsAg negative cases, since longitudinal studies and the detection of antibodies against hepatitis B viral antigens may reveal further associations. This phenomenon of liver positivity and sero-negativity has recently been confirmed in several groups of patients including haemophiliacs with only circulating anti-HBs (Spero et al., 1978).

In the 24 patients (including 5 with AHTC) with a histological diagnosis of acute hepatitis, HBsAg was found in 50% in the serum, and in 33% in the liver. These results of immunofluorescence and RIA in acute hepatitis are comparable to other observations (Edgington and Ritt, 1971; Mossor-Ostrowska et al., 1974). In particular, in the fully developed stage of acute hepatitis HBsAg was much more readily detectable in the serum than in the liver in contrast to the later stage of acute hepatitis and to AHTC in which HBsAg was detected in tissue and in serum, and to chronic hepatitis, in which HBsAg is more readily detectable in the tissue. These observations are consistent with the rare finding of HBsAg by immunofluorescence (Krawczynski et al., 1972; Gudat et al., 1975) and by electron microscopy (Nelson et al., 1970) in acute hepatitis. This supports the hypothesis that in acute hepatitis HBsAg-containing cells are cleared at high efficiency by normal immunological mechanisms (Dudley et al., 1972; Reed et al., 1974).

DISTRIBUTION PATTERNS OF HEPATITIS B SURFACE ANTIGEN IN THE LIVER OF HEPATITIS B PATIENTS

Acute and chronic viral hepatitis have distinct histological features (Desmet, 1970). In chronic hepatitis the amount of mononuclear cell infiltration in and around the portal tracts and the extent of liver cell damage indicate

55

the stage and severity of the disease. On the other hand predominant hepatocellular necrosis in the centrilobular area with less impressive portal infiltration plus accumulation of ceroid-containing macrophages, determine the stages of acute hepatitis (Bianchi *et al.*, 1971). Both acute and chronic hepatitis are found to be associated with infection with HBV (Blumberg *et al.*, 1967; Prince, 1968). The genesis of the diverse histological pictures is unknown – it has been postulated that this may be the result of variable host–virus interactions (Blumberg *et al.*, 1970; Dudley *et al.*, 1972). Based on this hypothesis one would expect at least some variation in the pattern of intrahepatic localization of HBsAg in various types of hepatitis B. In order to obtain some insight into this phenomenon and into the role played by HBV in the development of various types of hepatitis, a prospective immunofluorescence study was performed on the liver biopsies of 100 patients with both acute and chronic hepatitis.

Materials and methods

The 100 liver biopsies with the diagnosis of hepatitis included in the previous section were investigated in the present study.

Results

Of the 100 biopsies with histological diagnosis of hepatitis, 60 were positive for HBsAg: 52 cases of chronic hepatitis, 5 cases of acute hepatitis and 3 cases with AHTC. Of the 52 cases with chronic hepatitis, 40 had HBsAg in the serum and the remaining 12 were negative.

The distribution patterns of HBsAg in the hepatocytes were distinctive for both acute and chronic hepatitis. Four main expression patterns of HBsAg were obtained: full cytoplasmic fluorescence with diffuse lobular distribution; full or partial cytoplasmic positivity with spotty lobular distribution; peripheral fluorescence in the cell membrane and/or cell peripheries and focal cytoplasmic positivity. The results obtained with immunofluorescence are summarized in Table 3.4, and the individual characteristics of HBsAg expression in each histological type of hepatitis are described below.

Chronic persistent hepatitis

Approximately 60–70% of the hepatocytes were positive for HBsAg and the fluorescent cells were diffusely distributed throughout the liver lobules. The intensity of the fluorescence was strong and homogeneous in

56

Table 3.4 Summary of distribution pattern of HBsAg in acute and chronic hepatitis*

Histological diagnosis	Immunofluorescence positive	Diffuse lobular distribution	Scattered lobular distribution	Diffuse cytoplasmic, membrane and/or cell periphery	Focal cytoplasmic distribution
Chronic persistent hepatitis	6	3	1	1	2+
Chronic aggressive hepatitis	14	1	11	9	2+
Cirrhosis with little activity	5	3	—	—	2+
Active cirrhosis	27	5	15	15	6+ + 1
Acute hepatitis with signs of possible transition to chronicity	3	—	1	2	—
Fully developed stage of acute hepatitis, later and residual stage of acute hepatitis	5	—	—	—	5

* In cases with more than one distribution pattern, the numbers were put accordingly.
Biopsies from patients negative for circulating HBsAg

appearance (Figure 3.1). Of the 6 positive biopsies, 4 showed diffuse homogeneous cytoplasmic positivity; one of them showed positivity in the liver cell membranes extending over a significant part of cell periphery. The remaining two biopsies from serum negative patients showed specific fluorescence restricted to only a small part of the cytoplasm (focal cytoplasmic fluorescence).

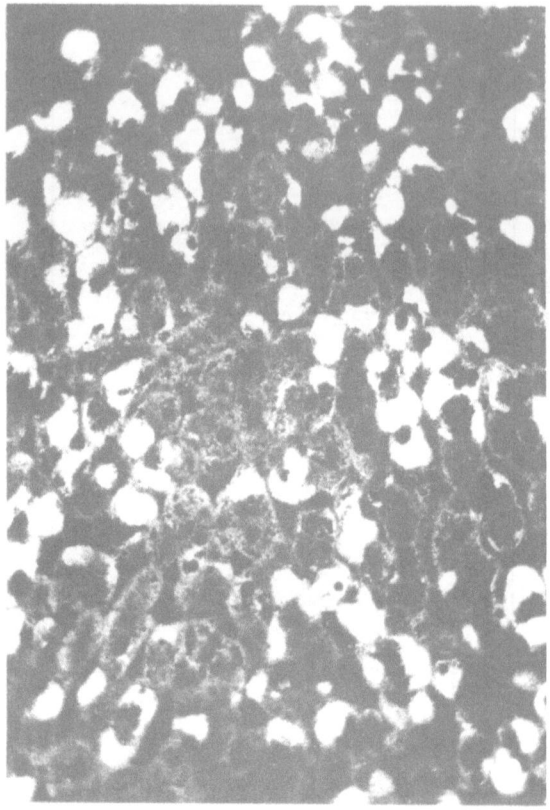

Figure 3.1 Chronic persistent hepatitis: HBsAg fluorescence is strong and homogeneous and positive cells are diffusely distributed within the lobules (× 230)

Chronic aggressive hepatitis

In CAH, cytoplasmic positivity was scattered throughout the lobule. At the cellular level, the fluorescence was predominantly found in the liver cell membranes and sometimes encroached on part of the liver cell periphery. The number of cytoplasmic positive cells was less than in CPH.

On most occasions, intracellular fluorescence was confined to only part of the fluorescence found in CPH and less active cirrhosis. The cytoplasmic fluorescence was dense and homogeneous in character. The intensity of the fluorescence in the cell membranes and in the cell periphery was strong and mostly granular. Intense fluorescence was restricted mainly to the sinusoidal pole of the hepatocytes. Of the 14 positive biopsies, 11 showed scattered cytoplasmic positivity. Nine of these 11 had membrane-localized HBsAg. Two biopsies from serum negative patients showed focal cytoplasmic fluorescence.

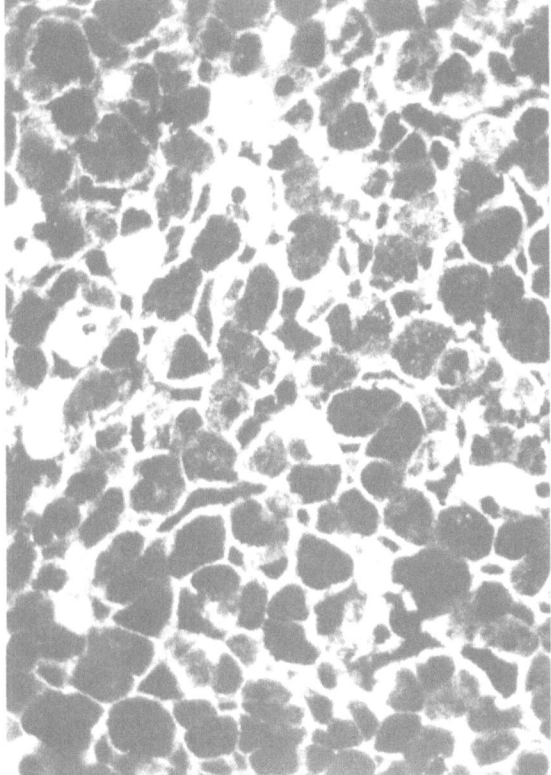

Figure 3.2 Chronic aggressive hepatitis: HBsAg is predominantly observed in the cell membrane and/or cell periphery. Only a few hepatocytes show partial or full cytoplasmic positivity ($\times$ 230)

Less active cirrhosis

The distribution pattern of HBsAg observed in less active cirrhosis was almost the same as that of CPH. Diffuse homogeneous fluorescence was present in 80–90% of the hepatocytes in the cirrhotic nodule (Figure 3.3). In some biopsies, positive cells were present in one part of the biopsy but no positive cells were found in the other. The intensity of fluorescence was strong. Three of the five positive biopsies showed diffuse cytoplasmic fluorescence and the remaining two from serum negative cases only had focal cytoplasmic positivity. No specific fluorescence was detected in the liver cell membrane.

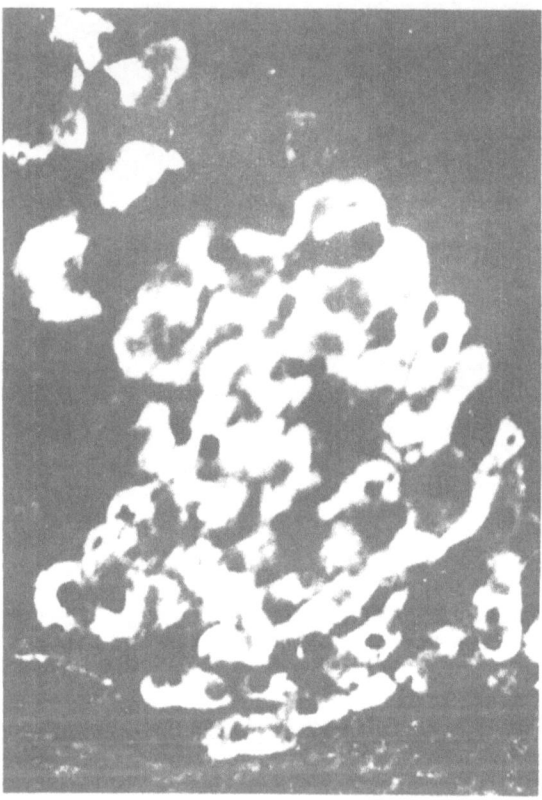

Figure 3.3 Less active cirrhosis: HBsAg is present in the cell cytoplasm distributed diffusely in a cirrhotic nodule (× 230)

Active cirrhosis

In active cirrhosis the number of positive cells was lower than in the less active form but higher than in CAH. The positive cells were distributed unevenly in the cirrhotic nodules. The fluorescence was granular and of low intensity, in contrast to the strong immunofluorescence observed in CAH (Figure 3.4). Membrane-localized HBsAg was also observed. Occasionally the fluorescence appeared to be thinly spread all over the hepatocytic cytoplasm. Of the 27 positive biopsies, 15 showed scattered positivity and all of them had membrane localized HBsAg. Seven biopsies, six of them from seronegative patients, showed focal cytoplasmic positivity (Figure 3.5). Only five of the positive biopsies showed diffuse cytoplasmic fluorescence without cell membrane positivity.

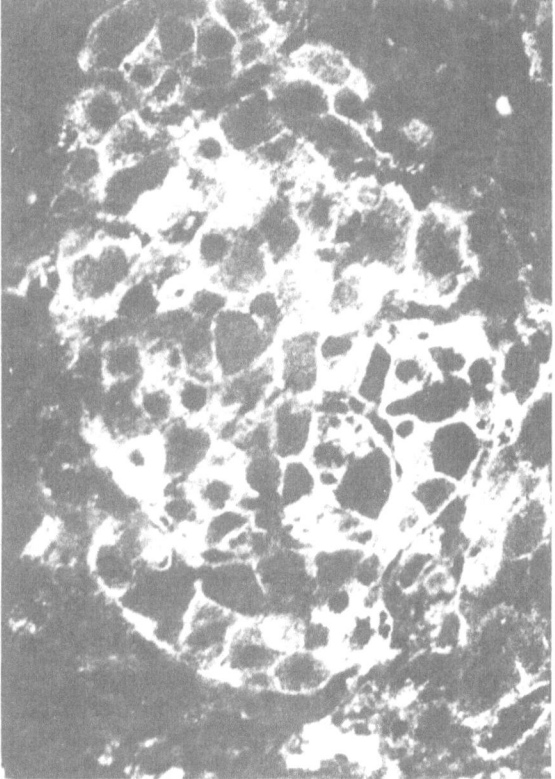

Figure 3.4 Active cirrhosis: HBsAg is demonstrated both in the cell membrane and in the cytoplasm of the hepatocytes. The fluorescence is moderate to low in intensity but the number of cells showing cytoplasmic positivity is higher compared with chronic aggressive hepatitis (× 230)

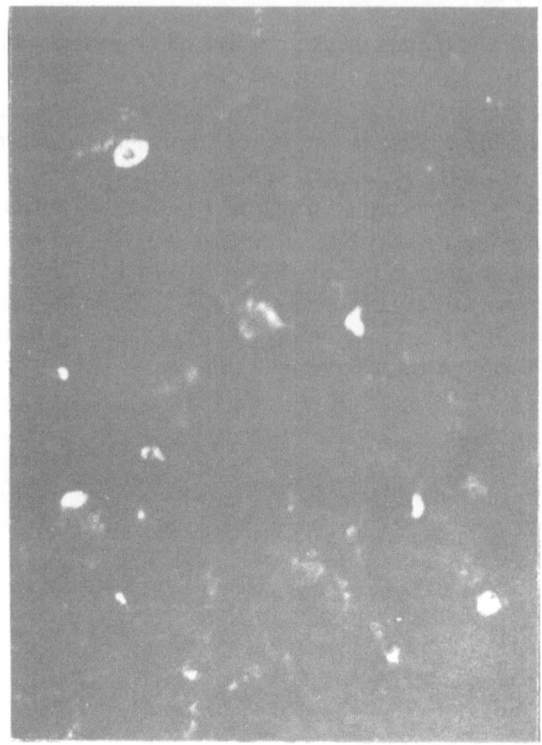

Figure 3.5 Biopsy of a patient with active cirrhosis without circulating HBsAg. Specific fluorescence is restricted to a part of the hepatocytic cytoplasm (focal cytoplasmic distribution) (× 230)

Acute hepatitis with possible signs of transition to chronicity

In this group of biopsies, HBsAg was demonstrated predominantly in the cell membrane of the hepatocytes as in CAH. However, the number of cytoplasmic positive cells was lower in comparison to CAH (Figure 3.6). The fluorescence was strong and mostly granular in character. In two of the three positive biopsies only the cell membrane HBsAg was observed. The remaining single biopsy showed a rare positive cell without membrane fluorescence.

Acute hepatitis

In fully developed acute hepatitis, HBsAg was rarely detected in the liver despite its presence in the serum. When present, mostly in later and

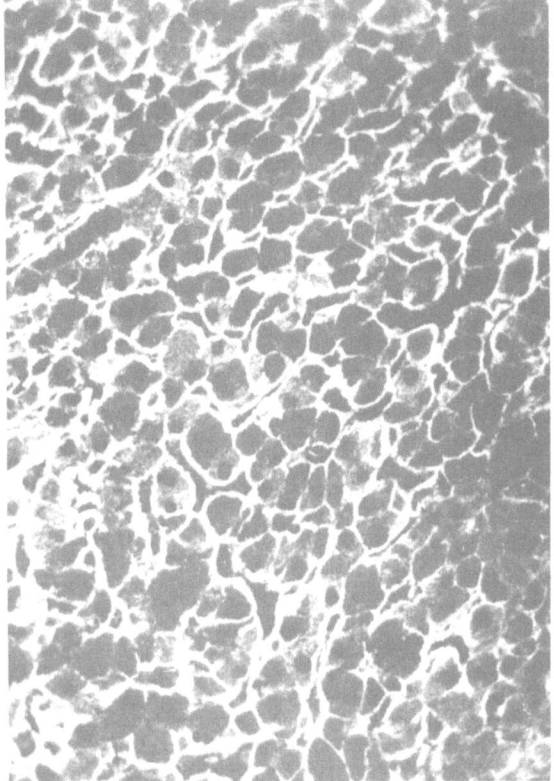

Figure 3.6 Acute hepatitis with signs of possible transition to chronicity. HBsAg is observed mainly in the cell membrane. Rarely the antigen is demonstrated in the hepato-cytic cytoplasm (× 230)

residual stages, the amount of antigen was very low. In the five positive biopsies the HBsAg was found either in the perinuclear area or localized focally in the cytoplasm.

Discussion

The present investigation revealed distinct intrahepatic distribution patterns of HBsAg in acute and chronic hepatitis B. An abundant amount of antigen present both at the cellular and lobular level characterizes CPH and less active cirrhosis. Moreover there is striking absence or only a minimal amount of membrane-localized HBsAg in those cases. On the other hand, fewer cells with cytoplasmic HBsAg with scattered cell positivity is characteristic of CAH, active cirrhosis and AHTC in which cases liver cell necrosis is more prominent. The membrane-localized HBsAg is a predominant feature in these conditions. In acute hepatitis and in the group of positive biopsies of patients with chronic hepatitis, whose serum was negative for HBsAg, the amount of antigen was low and showed a focal cytoplasmic localization. This inverse relationship between the amount of HBsAg in the liver and hepatocellular necrosis is shown schematically in Figure 3.7.

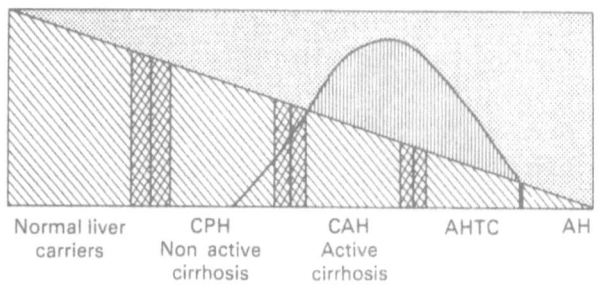

| Normal liver carriers | CPH Non active cirrhosis | CAH Active cirrhosis | AHTC | AH |

▢ NECROSIS

▨ FLUORESCENT CELLS

▥ CELL MEMBRANE & CELL PERIPHERY

Figure 3.7 Intrahepatic expression patterns of HBsAg and its relation to hepatocellular necrosis. High amount of HBsAg is present in non-aggressive group, i.e. in normal HBsAg carriers, CPH and in less active cirrhosis compared to the aggressive group, i.e. CAH, active cirrhosis and in AHTC. HBsAg is absent or rarely demonstrable in acute hepatitis. Membrane-localized HBsAg is mostly present in aggressive group of hepatitis

The described patterns of HBsAg may be the result of variation in host–virus interactions (Blumberg *et al.*, 1970; Dudley *et al.*, 1972; Reed *et al.*, 1974). The presence of large amount of antigen in CPH and less active cirrhosis may be due to the inadequate clearance of the antigen by the specific immunological defence system of the host. The absence of membrane-localized HBsAg may prevent these cells from becoming target cells for the immune response. On the other hand in CAH, active cirrhosis and AHTC the amount of antigen is low in the liver. In these instances, the immune system is efficient enough to clear most but not all antigen from the liver. The presence of membrane-localized HBsAg, however, renders these cells recognizable as target cells for the immune system resulting in cellular necrosis and antigen elimination.

In acute hepatitis very little or no antigen was detected in the liver by the immunofluorescence technique used in this study. This confirms other works performed both by immunofluorescence (Krawczynski *et al.*, 1972;

Cérat et al., 1973; Gudat et al., 1975) and electron microscopy (Nelson et al., 1970; Caramia et al., 1972). It also supports the hypothesis that the antigen or antigen-containing hepatocytes are completely cleared by a normally functioning specific immune system. (Dudley et al., 1972).

There is a remarkable correlation between the histological feature of 'piecemeal necrosis' (periportal hepatitis) (Ray et al., 1976b) and membrane-localized HBsAg. Both occur in CAH, active cirrhosis and AHTC. This finding suggests a relationship between liver cell membrane expression of HBsAg and the intralobular infiltration of mononuclear cells, supposed to be immunologically competent cells.

The focal intracellular presence of HBsAg in seronegative patients may reflect intrahepatocytic presence of HBsAg without actual release of viral components into the blood. These findings indicate that immunofluorescence detection of HBsAg in the liver biopsy may be a more dependable technique for sorting out 'carriers' of HBV than the search for HBsAg in the serum even with RIA. On the other hand it may be postulated that this group of patients is on the verge of clearing the antigen from the blood but has not yet completely cleared it from the liver. This phenomenon of an earlier clearance of HBsAg from the serum than from the liver has been observed during induction of experimental hepatitis in chimpanzees (Chapter 7).

The rare hepatocytes containing focal intracellular HBsAg in patients with acute hepatitis (supposed to have an adequate immune response for the clearance of HBV) may represent the remaining positive liver cells which escaped destruction during the necrotizing episode of fully developed acute hepatits; the HBsAg was not expressed at the cell's periphery and hence they were not recognized as possible target cells. Continuing HBsAg production and subsequent expression at the cell's periphery may be the mechanism involved in repeated attacks of relapsing hepatitis. This hypothesis would also imply that membrane expression of HBsAg in the liver cells has occurred before the necrotizing episode of acute hepatitis. Although biopsies from patients in the incubation period were not available, our own observations (Chapter 7) and the work done by Barker et al (1973) in experimental hepatitis B in chimpanzees indicate the presence of membrane-localized HBsAg before the onset of overt hepatitis. A recent investigation on isolated hepatocytes obtained from patients in the incubation period of hepatitis B shows HBsAg in the hepatocytic membrane (Alberti et al., 1976).

Finally, it is evident that HBsAg is expressed differently in the liver of patients with hepatitis B in its various clinicopathological manifestations; taking into account all the distinct expression patterns, it may be possible to refine the histological diagnosis on liver biopsies.

HEPATITIS B VIRUS ANTIGENS IN TISSUES

References

Alberti, A., Realdi, G., Tremolada, F. and Spina, G. P. (1976). Liver cell surface localization of hepatitis B antigen and of immunoglobulins in acute and chronic hepatitis and in liver cirrhosis. *Clin. Exp. Immunol.*, **25**, 396

Barker, L. F., Chisari, F. U., McGrath, P. P., Dalgard, D. W., Kirschstein, R. L., Almeida, J. D., Edgington, T. S., Sharp, G. D. and Peterson, M. R. (1973). Transmission of viral hepatitis type B to chimpanzees. *J. Infect. Dis.*, **127**, 648

Bianchi, L., De Groote, J., Desmet, V. J., Gedigk, P., Korb, G., Popper, H., Poulsen, H., Scheuer, P., Schmid, M., Thaler, H. and Wepler, W. (1971). Morphological criteria in viral hepatitis. *Lancet*, **1**, 333

Bianchi, P., Bianchi, P. C., Coltori, M., Dardanoni, L., Del Veechio-blanco, C., Fagiolo, U., Farini, R., Menozzi, I., Naccarato, R., Pagliaro, L., Spanò, C. and Verme, G. (1972). Occurrence of Australia antigen in chronic hepatitis in Italy. *Gastroenterology*, **63**, 482

Blumberg, B. S., Gerstley, B. J. S., Hungerford, D. A., London, W. T. and Sutnick, A. I. (1967). A serum antigen (Australia antigen) in Down's syndrome, leukaemia and hepatitis. *Ann. Int. Med.*, **66**, 924

Blumberg, B. S., Sutnick, A. I. and London, W. T. (1970). Australia antigen as a hepatitis virus. Variation in host response. *Am. J. Med.*, **48**, 1

Bulkley, B. H., Heizer, W. D., Goldfinger, S. E., Isselbacher, K. J. and Shulman, N. R. (1970). Distinctions in chronic active hepatitis based on circulating hepatitis-associated antigen. *Lancet*, **2**, 1323

Caramia, F., De Bac, C. and Ricci, G. (1972). Virus-like particles within hepatocytes of Australia antigen carriers. *Am. J. Dis. Child.*, **123**, 309

Cérat, G., Richer, G., Viallet, A., Côté, J., Robert, J. and Turgeon, F. (1973). Detection of Australia antigen in liver biopsies by immunofluorescence. *Canad. Med. Ass. J.*, **108**, 981

Cooksley, W. G. E., Pawell, L. W., Mistilis, S. P., Olsen, G., Mathews, J. D. and Mackay, I. R. (1972). Australia antigen in active chronic hepatitis in Australia: results in 130 patients from three centers. *Aust. NZ J. Med.*, **3**, 261

Cooksley, W. G. E., Powell, L. W., Mistilis, S. P., Mackay, I. R. and Barker, L. F. (1975). Hepatitis B antigen and antibody in active chronic hepatitis and other liver diseases in Australia. *Am. J. Dig. Dis.*, **20**, 110

Coyne (Zavatone), V. E., Millman, I., Cerda, J., Gerstley, B. J. S., London, T., Sutnick, A. and Blumberg, B. S. (1970). Localization of Australia antigen by immunofluorescence. *J. Exp. Med.*, **131**, 307

Desmet, V. J. (1970). Histopathology of acute and chronic hepatitis. In S. Gorini and D. Mori (ed.). *The Chronic Hepatitis*, Proceedings of the International Course in Hepatology. pp. 7–23. (Milan: Fondazione, Giovanni Lorenzini)

Dudley, F. J., Fox, R. A. and Sherlock, S. (1972). Cellular immunity and hepatitis-associated Australia antigen in liver disease. *Lancet*, **1**, 723

Edgington, T. S. and Ritt, D. J. (1971). Intrahepatic expression of serum hepatitis virus-associated antigens. *J. Exp. Med.*, **134**, 871

Gudat, F., Bianchi, L., Sonnabend, W., Thiel, G., Aenishaenslin, W. and Stalder, G. A. (1975). Pattern of core and surface expression in liver tissue reflects state of specific immune response in hepatitis B. *Lab. Invest.*, **32**, 1

Hadziyannis, S., Vissoulis, Ch., Moussouros, A. and Afroudakis, A. (1972). Cytoplasmic localization of Australia antigen in the liver. *Lancet*, **1**, 976

66

Krawczynski, K., Nazarewicz, T., Brzosko, W. J. and Nowoslawski, A. (1972). Cellular localization of hepatitis-associated antigen in livers of patients with different forms of hepatitis. *J. Infect. Dis.*, **126**, 372

Ling, C. M. and Overby, L. R. (1972). Prevalence of hepatitis B virus antigen as revealed by direct radioimmunoassay with ^{125}I-antibody. *J. Immunol.*, **109**, 834

Mason, E. C., Shaw, A. E., Harding, M. J. and Witney, K. J. (1972). High-voltage immunoelectroosmophoresis in Australia antigen screening of blood donors. *Med. J. Aust.*, **1**, 1020

Mossor-Ostrowska, J., Sowa, J. and Nazarewicz, T. (1974). Auto-antibodies in the serum and Australia antigen both in the serum and in tissue in diseases of the liver (Abstract). In Proceedings of 6th International Congress of Infectious Diseases, p. 100. (Warsaw: Academy of Medicine)

Nelson, J. M., Berker, L. F. and Danovitch, S. H. (1970). Intranuclear aggregates in the liver of a patient with serum hepatitis. *Lancet*, **2**, 773

Popper, H. and Schaffner, F. (1971). The vocabulary of chronic hepatitis. *N. Engl. J. Med.*, **284**, 1154

Prince, A. M. (1968). An antigen detected in the blood during the incubation period of serum hepatitis. *Proc. Nat. Acad. Sci. USA*, **60**, 814

Prince, A. M. (1971). Role of serum hepatitis virus in chronic liver disease. *Gastroenterology*, **60**, 913

Prince, A. M., Hargrove, R. L., Szmuness, W., Cherubin, C. E., Fontana, V. J. and Jeffries, G. H. (1970). Immunologic distinction between infectious and serum hepatitis. *N. Engl. J. Med.*, **282**, 987

Ray, M. B., Desmet, V. J., Fevery, J., De Groote, J., Bradburne, A. F. and Desmyter, J. (1976a). Hepatitis B surface antigen in the liver of patients with hepatitis: a comparison with serological detection. *J. Clin. Path.*, **29**, 89

Ray, M. B., Desmet, V. J., Fevery, J., De Groote, J., Bradburne, A. F. and Desmyter, J. (1976b). Distribution patterns of hepatitis B surface antigen (HBsAg) in the liver of hepatitis patients. *J. Clin. Path.*, **29**, 94

Reed, W. D., Eddleston, A. L. W. F., Stern, R. B., Williams, R., Zuckerman, A. J., Bowes, A. and Earl, P. M. (1973). Detection of hepatitis B antigen by radioimmunoassay in chronic liver disease and hepatocellular carcinoma in Great Britain. *Lancet*, **2**, 690

Reed, W. D., Eddleston, A. L. W. F. and Williams, R. (1974). Immunopathology of viral hepatitis in man. *Progr. Med. Virol.*, **17**, 38

Sherlock, S., Fox, R. A., Niazi, S. P. and Scheuer, P. J. (1970). Chronic liver disease and primary liver-cell cancer with hepatitis-associated (Australia) antigen in serum. *Lancet*, **1**, 1243

Shulman, N. R. and Barker, L. F. (1969). Virus-like antigen, antibody, and antigen–antibody complexes in hepatitis measured by complement fixation. *Science*, **165**, 304

Skinhoj, P., Nielsen, J. O. and Dietrichson, O. (1977). Serological evidence of hepatitis B infection in patients with chronic liver disease: radioimmunoassay of HBsAg and anti-HBs. *Scand. J. Gastroent.*, **12**, 615

Spero, J. A., Lewis, J. H., Vanthiel, D. H., Hasiba, U. and Rabin, B. S. (1978). Asymptomatic structural liver disease in haemophilia. *N. Engl. J. Med.*, **298**, 1373

Sutnick, A. I., London, W. T. and Blumberg, B. S. (1969). Australia antigen and the quest for a hepatitis virus. *Am. J. Dig. Dis.*, **14**, 189

Velasco, M. and Katz, R. (1970). Hepatitis-associated antigen in chronic liver disease. *Lancet*, **1**, 779

Wenzel, R. P., Teates, C. D., Querido Galapon, R. T., Barczak, R., Ling, C. M. and Overby, L. R. (1975). Acute viral hepatitis in adults. *JAMA*, **232,** 366

Wewalka, F., Gnan, F., Krassnitsky, O. and Pesendorfer, F. (1970). Au/SH-antigen in liver disease. *Vox Sang. (Basel),* **19,** 311

Wright, R. (1970). The Australia antigen in chronic active hepatitis. *Vox Sang. (Basel),* **19,** 320

4
Intrahepatic expression patterns of hepatitis B surface and hepatitis B core antigen in the liver of hepatitis B patients

The core and surface proteins of HBV have entirely different antigenic specifications (Almeida *et al.*, 1971; Huang and Groh, 1973; Barker *et al.*, 1974) and can be visualized in the liver mainly by immunofluorescence and electron microscopy (Gudat *et al.*, 1975). In the expectation of obtaining different expressions of HBcAg and HBsAg in various histological types of hepatitis B, the present study investigates the cellular localization of HBcAg along with HBsAg in patients with both acute and chronic hepatitis.

Materials and methods

One hundred frozen liver needle biopsies were included in this investigation. Of them, 70 biopsies were studied new and 30 were reprocessed from the 100 biopsies reported in the previous Chapter (3). The patients with a diagnosis of CAH or active cirrhosis were treated with prednisolone 15 mg daily with or without azathioprine 1 mg/kg of body weight per day systemically. Untreated patients are those whose biopsies were taken before this treatment was initiated.

The positive reactions obtained for HBs and HBc antigens were graded on a numerical scale. When less than 20% of the hepatocytes were positive the biopsy was graded 1 +. Between 20 and 50% positive cells were graded 2 + and more than 50% as 3+. It was unusual to observe 100% positive hepatocytes.

Results

Demonstration of HBsAg and HBcAg

The usual intracellular sites of location of HBsAg and HBcAg were described in Chapter 2 and the different expression patterns of HBsAg in liver biopsies from patients with hepatitis B were detailed in Chapter 3.

Relative proportions of HBcAg and HBsAg in different types of hepatitis

Of the 100 biopsies, 82 were from patients with different forms of chronic hepatitis and 14 were diagnosed as acute hepatitis in different stages of development. Biopsies from 4 patients were diagnosed as 'near normal liver'. The histological diagnosis and the results of immunofluorescence for both HBsAg and HBcAg and for circulating HBsAg are given in Table 4.1 and Figure 4.1.

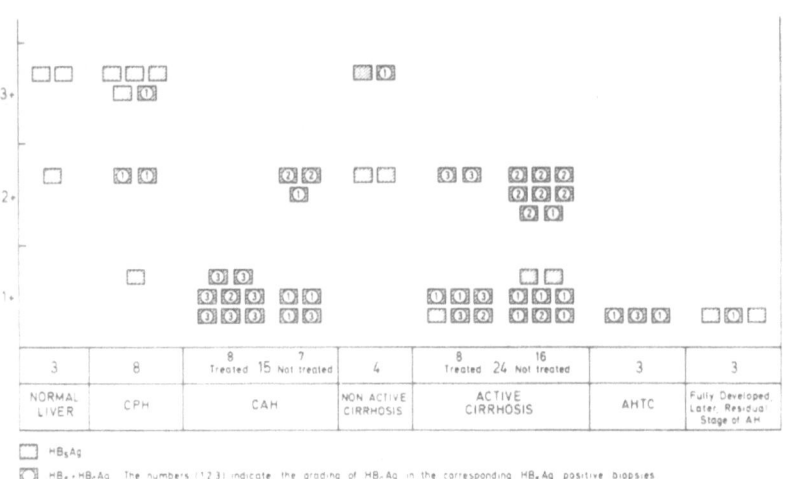

Figure 4.1   Relative proportions of intrahepatic HBsAg and HBcAg in hepatitis B antigens positive liver disease. HBsAg is more abundant in non-aggressive group than in aggresssive group of hepatitis B. HBcAg is most prevalent (3 +) in patients treated with immuno-suppressive agents

70

Table 4.1 Summary of distribution patterns of HBsAg and HBcAg in blood and liver of acute and chronic hepatitis

Histological diagnosis	Nos.	HBsAg+ blood	HBsAg + Liver				HBcAg + Liver			Ground-glass hepatocytes
			Cytoplasm	Grade	Membrane/cell periphery	Grade	Nucleus	Grade	Cytoplasm	
1. CHRONIC HEPATITIS										
(a) Chronic persistent hepatitis	12	8	8	+to+++	3	+to+	3	+	—	+to+++
(b) Chronic aggressive hepatitis	21	15	15	+to+++	15	++to+++	15	+to+++	2	+to++
(c) Cirrhosis with little activity	14	4	4	++to+++	1	+	1	+	—	+to++
(d) Active cirrhosis	35	21	24	+to++	19	+to+++	21	+to+++	2	+to++
Total	82	48	51		38		40		4	
2. ACUTE HEPATITIS										
(a) Fully developed stage of acute hepatitis	5	2	1	+	—	—	1	+	—	—
(b) Later stage of acute hepatitis	4	2	2	+	—	—	—	—	—	—
(c) Residual stage of acute hepatitis	1	—	—	—	—	—	—	—	—	—
3. ACUTE HEPATITIS WITH SIGNS OF POSSIBLE TRANSITION TO CHRONICITY	4	3	3	+	3	++to+++	3	+to+++	—	—
4. NORMAL LIVER	4	3	3	++to+++	—	—	—	—	—	++to+++
TOTAL	100	58	60		41		44		4	

Relation between membrane-localized HBsAg and nuclear HBcAg

In chronic hepatitis, 48 patients had circulating HBsAg whereas 51 were positive in the liver. In 38 of them HBsAg was localized in the cell membrane and/or periphery of the hepatocytes. The intensity of the membrane fluorescence and the number of membrane-positive cells were higher in active forms than in less active forms of chronic hepatitis (Table 4.1). HBcAg could be visualized in the liver of 40 patients. The frequency was higher in CAH (15 of 15) and active cirrhosis (21 of 24) than in CPH (3 of 8) and less active cirrhosis (1 of 4). All 38 biopsies positive for HBsAg in the cell membranes were also positive for HBcAg. However, in two biopsies of active cirrhosis no membrane positivity was observed although HBcAg was present.

In acute hepatitis 4 had circulating HBsAg and 3 of them were positive in the liver (1 fully developed stage, 2 later stage). In the fully developed and later stages, focal cytoplasmic positivity was obtained and no membrane-localized HBsAg was found. In one of five biopsies of fully developed acute hepatitis an occasional nucleus was found to be HBcAg positive. No HBcAg was observed in later stages of acute hepatitis.

In AHTC, 3 biopsies were positive for membrane-localized HBsAg and all of them had variable amounts of nuclear HBcAg.

HBsAg was detected both in the serum and in the liver of 3 of 4 patients with 'near normal liver'. There was no HBsAg in the cell membranes and HBcAg was not detectable.

Influence of treatment with immunosuppressive drugs on relative proportions of HBcAg and HBsAg

Of the 51 patients with chronic hepatitis with HBsAg in the liver, 16 (CAH – 8; active cirrhosis – 8) were treated with immunosuppressive drugs at variable doses and/or different lengths of time before the biopsies were taken. These biopsies showed more positive nuclei for HBcAg and a less cytoplasmic HBsAg in comparison to non-treated patients in the same group. Figure 4.1 illustrates the effect of immunosuppressive agents on the relative proportion of HBsAg and HBcAg.

In CAH, 7 of the 8 biopsies from treated patients showed 3 + HBcAg and 1 + HBsAg, whereas in the non-treated group only one had 3 + HBcAg and 1 + HBsAg. Five of the 6 remaining patients showed an equal balance between HBcAg and HBsAg.

In the group of active cirrhosis, 8 patients were treated with immuno-suppressive agents. Seven were HBcAg positive, 4 of these 7 had 3 + core, both of them had no membrane-localized HBsAg and both cases were positive (1 +), these two patients were both biochemically and histologically in the later stage of acute exacerbation of the illness. One of the treated patient was core negative and had faint cytoplasmic HBsAg without any membrane positivity; clinically and histologically this case was highly active. The non-treated group comprised 16 biopsies, 14 of them were positive both for HBsAg and HBcAg, 12 of these 14 had an equal balance of HBsAg and HBcAg. Two biopsies were negative for core, both of them had no membrane-localized HBsAg and both cases were active.

In the patients negative for HBsAg in the biopsy (CAH – 5; active cirrhosis – 11), no HBcAg was observed, although some of them received immunosuppressive drugs.

Patients with acute hepatitis, patients with a first biopsy establishing chronic hepatitis and patients with 'near normal liver' received no immunosuppressive drugs before biopsy.

HBsAg, ground glass hepatocytes and hepatocellular damage

HBsAg was abundant both at the cellular and lobular level in cases of near normal liver, CPH and less active cirrhosis; in all these groups liver cell necrosis and mononuclear cell infiltration is minimal. Most of these biopsies showed 3 + HBsAg fluorescence in the liver. This correlated well with the number of ground glass hepatocytes observed in the biopsies of those patients (Table 4.1). In contrast, the amount of both HBsAg and ground glass cells was low in case of CAH and active cirrhosis where the amount of hepatocellular necrosis and mononuclear cell infiltration was high. No ground glass hepatocytes were found in various stages of acute hepatitis.

Cytoplasmic localization of HBcAg

HBcAg was observed in the cytoplasm of hepatocytes only in 4 cases: 2 CAH and 2 active cirrhosis. Three of these 4 patients received immunosuppressive drugs before biopsy. The amount and distribution pattern of HBcAg in the liver cell cytoplasm of all four patients appeared similar irrespective of therapy.

Discussion

This immunofluorescence study revealed HBcAg mostly in the nuclei of the hepatocytes and rarely (4 cases) in the cytoplasm, whereas HBsAg was demonstrated in the cytoplasm and in the cell membranes of the hepatocytes. In HBsAg carriers, CPH and less active cirrhosis there was prominent expression of cytoplasmic HBsAg both by immunoflurescence and light microscopy (ground glass hepatocytes) whereas HBcAg and membrane-localized HBsAg were rarely observed. In acute hepatitis the amount of HBcAg and HBsAg both in the cytoplasm and in membranes was minimal or absent. In non-treated cases of CAH and active cirrhosis, and in AHTC, the balance between HBcAg and cytoplasmic HBsAg was almost equal but membrane-bound HBsAg was prominent. In treated cases of CAH and active cirrhosis there was a high amount of HBcAg and prominent membrane expression of HBsAg in comparison to cytoplasmic HBsAg.

An important observation is the correlation between HBsAg in the liver cell membranes and HBcAg in the nuclei. HBsAg expression in the liver cell membrane was mostly present in CAH and active cirrhosis (irrespective of immunosuppressive therapy) and in AHTC. In all of these conditions there is also prominent expression of HBcAg. The direct correlation between membrane-localized HBsAg and nuclear HBcAg is summarized in Figure 4.2. On the other hand HBsAg was not detectable in the liver cell membranes in 3 cases of active cirrhosis (all of which were highly active; one was treated) and no HBcAg was observed.

Furthermore, in CPH and less active cirrhosis, HBcAg positive nuclei were observed only in very small numbers in those cases where membrane-localized HBsAg was present. In near normal livers with ground glass hepatocytes there was no membrane-localized HBsAg and no HBcAg was detectable. It seems therefore that HBsAg in the hepatocyte membrane and HBcAg in the nuclei is related to immunological activity of the disease process, apparently indicating continuous viral replication and release with eventual formation of Dane particles. This idea can be substantiated by the presence of abundant Dane particles in the serum of patients with

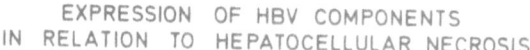

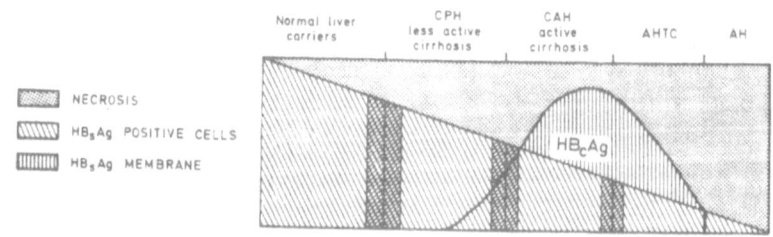

Figure 4.2 Shows direct correlation between membrane-localized HBsAg and nuclear HBcAg. Both antigens are predominantly present in aggressive group of hepatitis B

74

CAH as compared with healthy carriers (Nielsen *et al.*, 1973; Woolf *et al.*, 1975).

The direct correlation between the presence of membrane-localized HBsAg and periportal (piecemeal) necrosis, the probable recognition and subsequent elimination of antigen-containing hepatocytes (target cells) by the specific immune system has been discussed in Chapter 3.

In patients receiving immunosuppressive drugs there is a higher number of HBcAg positive nuclei as compared to HBsAg-containing cells. These results are similar to those obtained in kidney transplant patients by Gudat *et al.* (1975). Apparently the present series of patients studied is different in that they received therapy after the onset of hepatitis whereas the patients with renal transplants may have received the therapy before the initiation of infection by HBV. Moreover they received prednisolone with or without azathioprine in low dosage, the immunosuppressive effect of which may be doubted. Similar results of HBcAg predominance were reported by electron microscopy in cases with malignant lymphoma (Nowoslawsky *et al.*, 1970) and patients with renal transplant (Huang *et al.*, 1974). The reasons for this HBcAg predominance in these patients is not clear. However, they may have a drug-induced suppression of specific immune systems needed to destroy and eliminate the affected cells. Recently it has been shown that corticosteroids inhibit the cytolytic activity of 'T' lymphocytes *in vitro* (Wands *et al.*, 1975).

HBcAg was demonstrated in the liver cell cytoplasm in active forms of chronic hepatitis B. These HBcAg-specific fluorescent granules may correspond to the non-coated virus-like particles, different from membrane-bound inclusions inside the endoplasmic reticulum (Stein *et al.*, 1971) and visualized in the cytoplasm of the hepatocytes by electron microscopy (Dunn *et al.*, 1972). The immunofluorescence demonstration of cytoplasmic HBcAg has recently been confirmed by several other groups (Gudat and Bianchi, 1977; Spero *et al.*, 1978). This observation lends support to the suggestion that Dane particles are assembled in the membrane of the hepatocytes.

In conclusion, it may be summarized that the various expressions of HBcAg and HBsAg at the cellular level and the ultimate development of different histological types of hepatitis maybe the result of an interaction between the HBV and the host's immune system.

References

Almeida, J. D., Rubenstein, D. and Stott, E. J. (1971). New antigen–antibody system in Australia-antigen-positive hepatitis. *Lancet*, 2, 1225

Barker, L. F., Almeida, J. D., Hoofnagle, J. H., Gerety, R. J., Jackson, R. and McGrath,

P. P. (1974). Hepatitis B core antigen: immunology and electron microscopy. *J. Virol*, **14**, 1552

Dunn, A. E. G., Peters, R. L., Schweitzer, I. L., Ivoin, L. and Spears, R. L. (1972). Virus-like particles in livers of infants with vertically transmitted hepatitis. *Arch. Path.*, **94**, 258

Gudat, F., Bianchi, L., Sonnabend, W., Thiel, G., Aenishaenslin, W. and Stalder, G. A. (1975). Pattern of core and surface expression in liver tissue reflects state of immune response in hepatitis B. *Lab. Invest.*, **32**, 1

Gudat, F. and Bianchi, L. (1977). Evidence for phasic sequences in nuclear HBsAg formation and cell membrane directed flow of core particles in chronic hepatitis B. *Gastroenterology*, **73**, 1194

Huang, S. and Groh, V. (1973). A study on antibodies produced with liver tissue containing Australia antigen and virus-like particles. *Lab. Invest.*, **29**, 743

Huang, S., Groh, V., Beaudoin, J. G., Dauphinee, W. D., Guttmann, R. D., Morehouse, D. D., Aronoff, A. and Gault, H. A. (1974). A study of the relationship of virus-like particles and Australia antigen in liver. *Hum. Path.*, **5**, 209

Nielsen, J. O., Nielsen, M. H. and Elling, P. (1973). Differential distribution of Australia-antigen-associated particles in patients with liver diseases and normal carriers. *N. Engl. J. Med.*, **288**, 484

Nowoslawsky, A., Brzosko, W. J. and Madalinski, K. (1970). Cellular localization of Australia antigen in the liver of patients with lympho proliferative disorders. *Lancet*, **1**, 494

Spero, J. A., Lewis, J. H., Van Thiel, D. H., Hasiba, U. and Rabin, B. S. (1978). Asymptomatic structural liver disease in haemophilia. *N. Engl. J. Med.*, **298**, 1373

Stein, O., Fainaru, M. and Stein, Y. (1971). Virus-like particles in cytoplasm of livers of Au-antigen carriers. *Lancet*, **2**, 90

Wands, J. R., Perrotto, J. L., Alpert, E. and Isselbacher, K. J. (1975). Cell-mediated immunity in acute and chronic hepatitis. *J. Clin. Invest.*, **55**, 921

Woolf, I. L., Jones, D. M., Tapp, E. and Dymock, I. W. (1975). Electron-microscopy of serum of healthy hepatitis B antigen carriers. *J. Clin. Path.*, **28**, 260

5
Hepatitis B core antigen immune complexes in the liver of hepatitis B patients

The distinctive localization patterns of HBsAg and HBcAg obtained in various types of hepatitis B were described in Chapter 4. The factors responsible for this distinctive expression of HBV components and the ultimate development of various histological types of hepatitis B remain obscure. Early studies supported the view that HBsAg immune complexes may mediate liver cell damage in hepatitis B (Nowoslawski *et al.*, 1972). This chapter deals with studies on humoral immune mechanisms and their possible role in the development of hepatitis B.

The present study investigates the localization patterns of HBsAg, HBcAg and various immunoglobulins and *in vitro* complement fixation in 102 liver specimens. The results obtained were correlated with the histological diagnosis and with circulating anti-HBs and anti-HBc (Ray *et al.*, 1979).

Materials and methods

One hundred and two frozen liver biopsies obtained from 102 clinically diagnosed hepatitis patients were included in this investigation. Of them, 60 were among 100 studied in Chapter 4. The remaining 42 specimens were new. Some patients of CAH and active cirrhosis received treatment similarly as mentioned in Chapter 4.

The present series of biopsies were examined in the same fluorescence microscope as mentioned previously but fitted with an additional XBO 75 lamp.

77

In vitro *complement fixation (VCF) and immunoglobulin*

The procedure of VCF was performed according to Burkholder (1961) using fresh human serum as complement source. Unfixed $4\,\mu m$ thick cryostat sections were incubated first with fresh human serum (obtained from donors of blood groups AB and negative for antinuclear factors, anti-HBc and anti-HBs) for 45 min at 37°C followed by RAHu/C3/FITC (FITC conjugated rabbit immunoglobulin G against human complement C3) for 30 min at the same temperature. Heat-inactivated (56 °C for 1 hour) fresh human serum (obtained from the same sources) was used as control. A serial section was also incubated with RAHu/C3/FITC alone. Serial sections were examined for IgG, IgA and IgM.

Double staining with contrast colour fluorochromes

To investigate the relationship between the cells containing HBV components and those with complement fixing capacity, two parallel sections of positive biopsies were incubated with FITC and TRITC conjugated specific antisera in the following sequence:

(a) Rabbit anti-HBs + GAR/TRITC + human anti-HBc/FITC
(b) Normal human serum + GAHu/C3/TRITC + human anti-HBc/FITC.

After each incubation step, slides were washed in PBS, mounted as usual and examined alternately in FITC and TRITC excitation wavelengths.

Serology

From 102 patients tested for HBsAg, sera from 88 were available for estimating both anti-HBs and anti-HBc.

Results

Demonstration of HBsAg and HBcAg in the liver biopsy

The intrahepatic distribution patterns of both HBsAg and HBcAg obtained in various histological types of hepatitis B were similar to those reported in Chapter 4.

Demonstration of in vitro *complement fixation in the liver biopsy*

Complement fixation was demonstrated in the nucleus and cytoplasm of the hepatocytes and observed as bright granular fluorescent dots. Most of the hepatocytes showed staining either in the nuclei or in the cytoplasm. Relatively few cells gave a specific reaction both in the nucleus and in the cytoplasm (Figure 5.1). Sometimes Kupffer cells were also positive.

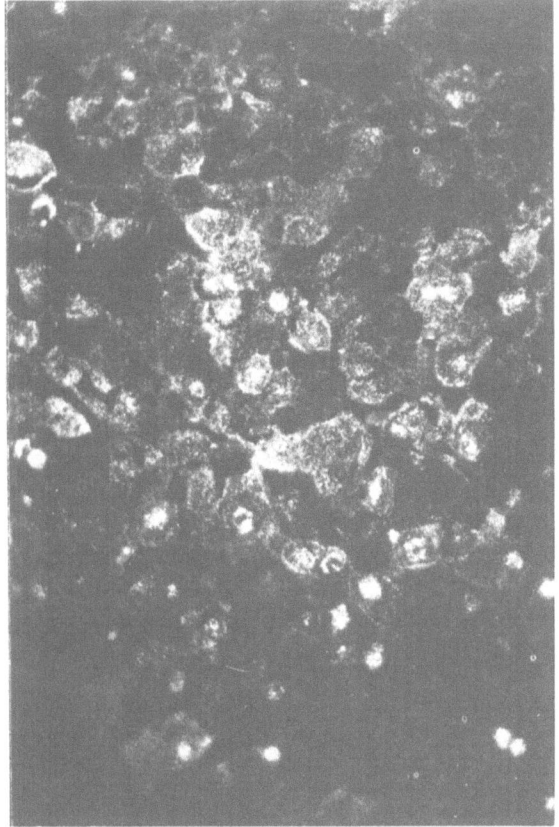

Figure 5.1 Liver biopsy from a patient with untreated CAH: *in vitro* complement fixation: positivity is present both in the nuclei and cytoplasm of the hepatocytes. Cytoplasmic complement fixation is coarse granular and is observed in the periphery of the hepatocytes (× 230)

This positive reaction was obtained only after incubation with fresh human serum followed by conjugated antihuman C3. No reaction was observed after treating the sections either with conjugated antihuman C3 alone or pre-incubating the specimens with heat-inactivated normal serum obtained from the same source.

Localization of immunoglobulins

The three immunoglobulin classes were mostly observed singly but also, rarely, in combination. IgG was observed alone in the hepatocytic nuclei of 90% of the biopsies positive for immunoglobulins. IgM was detected only

79

twice, each time along with IgG. IgA was seen only in one biopsy. In most instances, the fluorescence was granular and of variable intensity. Immunoglobulins were stained in the cytoplasm of the liver cells very faintly and rarely. Liver sinusoids were stained strongly especially with anti-IgG sera, preventing correct interpretation of the presence of IgG in the cell membranes. However, occasionally granular deposits of IgG were observed in the liver cell membranes.

Demonstration of HBV components by double staining procedures

After double staining of positive specimens for HBsAg and HBcAg, different combination patterns were found. Some liver cells only contained HBcAg in the nucleus; others were only positive for HBsAg either in the cytoplasm or in the cell membranes. However, a substantial proportion of liver cells expressed both antigens, especially when the cell membrane localization of HBsAg is taken into account. Cytoplasmic HBsAg was better visualized in the orange (rhodamine) background of HBsAg positivity. In sections containing HBcAg, after treatment with fresh human serum and double staining with antihuman C3/TRITC, HBcAg-containing nuclei were shown to fix C3. The number of VCF-positive cells was higher than that of HBcAg containing cells (Figures 5.2 and 5.3).

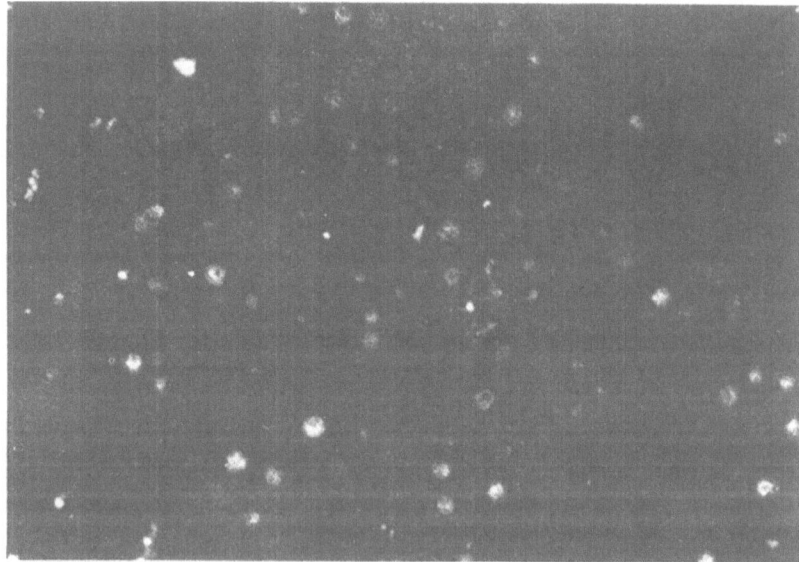

Figure 5.2 Biopsy from patient with untreated CAH: double stained: first with normal human serum followed by GAHu/C3/TRITC; then anti-HBc/FITC HBcAg specific green fluorescence is limited to hepatocytic nuclei (× 230)

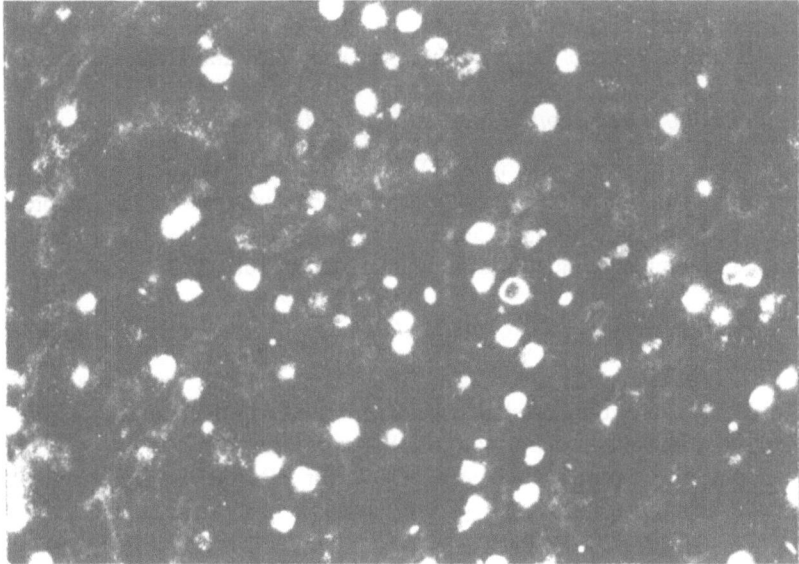

Figure 5.3 Same area as in Figure 5.2; photographed after adjusting the filters specific for TRITC: HBcAg positive nuclei are shown to fix complement *in vitro*. Moreover the red fluorescence is stronger and the number of complement positive nuclei is higher than the number of HBcAg positive nuclei (× 230)

Incidence of circulating anti-HBs and anti-HBc in hepatitis patients

Table 5.1 shows the frequencies of anti-HBs and anti-HBc both in HBsAg positive and HBsAg negative cases of acute and chronic hepatitis. In HBsAg seropositive chronic hepatitis, 85% (34 of 40 examined) had circulating anti-HBc and the remaining 15% (6 of 40) had both anti-HBs and anti-HBc in the blood. Therefore, in this group, 100% cases had circulating anti-HBc. In HBsAg negative chronic hepatitis 24% (6 of 25 examined) were positive for anti-HBc alone and 8% (2 of 25) were positive for both anti-HBc and anti-HBs. 12% (3 of 25) had only anti-HBs. In this HBsAg seronegative group only two patients with active cirrhosis had demonstrable HBsAg in the liver. They had no circulating anti-HBs but anti-HBc was present in the blood.

In HBsAg seropositive acute hepatitis 83% (5 of 6) had anti-HBc in the blood in contrast to only 20% (1 of 5) in HBsAg negative hepatitis. In the HBsAg positive group, no cases were positive either for both anti-HBs and anti-HBc or for anti-HBs alone.

In HBsAg positive AHTC, all 4 patients examined had circulating anti-

HBc and none had anti-HBs or both. In the AHTC group, the single HBsAg negative case had no anti-HBc and/or anti-HBs in the blood.

All HBsAg carriers ('near normal liver') had only anti-HBc in the blood.

Relation between membrane-localized HBsAg and HBcAg

In chronic hepatitis and in AHTC, the direct correlation between the membrane-localized HBsAg and nuclear HBcAg was reported in Chapter 4, and the same patterns of relation exist in this study. The results obtained in the present investigation are summarized in Table 5.2.

Relation between HBcAg in the liver cells and in vitro complement fixation

Table 5.2 shows the correlation between HBcAg in the hepatocytes, VCF and immunoglobulin deposition in HBsAg positive livers. In chronic hepatitis, out of 39 biopsies which were positive for HBcAg, 35 fixed complement in the hepatocytes (21 both in the nucleus and cytoplasm and 14 only in the nuclei). The frequency of VCF was higher in CAH (17 of 21, of which 19 had HBcAg) and in active cirrhosis (14 of 20, of which 15 were positive for HBcAg) than in CPH (3 of 9, of which 4 had HBsAg) and less active cirrhosis (1 of 3, of which 1 was HBcAg positive). Of the total 21 cases positive for VCF both in the cytoplasm and nuclei, 11 had HBcAg in the same two sites. In CPH the single case which was negative for VCF had only a couple of nuclei weakly positive for HBcAg. In CAH (2 cases) and active cirrhosis (1 case) 3 biopsies positive for HBcAg were negative for VCF.

Only in a single case of fully developed acute hepatitis there were rare nuclei to be found, faintly positive for VCF, although no HBcAg was observed in the liver cells. In AHTC, 3 cases were positive for VCF, all three had HBcAg in the liver.

HBcAg was not visualized in cases histologically diagnosed as 'near normal liver' and all were negative for VCF.

Relation between in vitro complement fixation, immunoglobulin deposition in the liver cells and circulating anti-HBc

In HBsAg-positive chronic hepatitis, 29 of 35 cases positive for VCF also revealed a deposition of immunoglobulin, mostly IgG in the nuclei of the hepatocytes (Table 5.2). Out of these 29 patients, blood from 23 was available for the estimation of both anti-HBs and anti-HBc (Table 5.1; cases are indicated in parentheses). Anti-HBc was detected in the sera of all 23, whereas only 5 had additionally detectable anti-HBs (one patient

Table 5.1 Incidence of anti-HBs and anti-HBc in chronic and acute hepatitis and in HBsAg carriers

Histological diagnosis	No.	HBsAg	HBsAg+ group anti-HBs+ anti-HBc+	HBsAg+ group anti-HBs+ anti-HBc-	Blood anti-HBs- anti-HBc+	No.	HBsAg- group anti-HBs+ anti-HBc+	HBsAg- group anti-HBs+ anti-HBc-	HBsAg- group anti-HBs- anti-HBc+
1. CHRONIC HEPATITIS									
Chronic persistent hepatitis	12	9	0/8	0/8	8(3)/8	3	0/3	0/3	1/3
Chronic aggressive hepatitis	26	21	4(3)/17	0/17	13(9)/17	5	1/5	1/5	1/5
Less active cirrhosis	10	3	1(1)/3	0/3	2/3	7	1/6	0/6	1/6
Active cirrhosis	32	18	1(1)/12	0/12	11(6)/12	14*	0/11	2/11	3/9
Total	80	51	6(5)/40 (15%)	0/40 (0%)	34(18)/40(85%)	29	2/25 (8%)	3/25 (12%)	6/25 (24%)
2. ACUTE HEPATITIS									
Fully developed acute hepatitis	5	3	0/3	0/3	3/3	2	0/2	0/2	0/2
Later and residual stages of acute hepatitis	7	3	0/3	0/3	2/3	4	1/3	0/3	1/3
Total	12	6	0/6 (0%)	0/6 (0%)	5/6 (83%)	6	1/5 (20%)	0/5 (0%)	1/5 (20%)
3. ACUTE HEPATITIS WITH SIGNS OF TRANSITION TO CHRONICITY	6	5	0/4	0/4	4(3)/4	1	0/1	0/1	0/1
4. NEAR NORMAL LIVER	4	4	0/4 (4%)	0/4 (0%)	4/4 (100%)	0	0	0	0
TOTAL	102	66	6/54 (11%)	0/54 (0%)	47/54 (87%)	36	3/31 (10%)	3/31 (10%)	5/31 (16%)

* 2 cases which are tissue positive but serum negative, positive only for anti-HBc
Cases in parenthesis are positive for immunoglobulin

Table 5.2 Summary of distribution patterns of HBsAg, HBcAg and VCF and deposition of immunoglobulins in acute and chronic hepatitis B and in normal carrier

Histological diagnosis	Blood HBs+	Liver HBsAg			Liver HBcAg		Liver C3 fixation		Immuno-globulin (Ig)+
		Membrane+ cytoplasm+	Membrane+ cytoplasm−	Membrane− cytoplasm+	Nucleus+ cytoplasm+	Nucleus+ cytoplasm−	Nucleus+ cytoplasm+	Nucleus+ cytoplasm−	
1. CHRONIC HEPATITIS									
(1) Chronic persistent hepatitis	9	4	—	5[a,b,c]	1	3(2+1[b,c])	1	2	3
(2) Chronic aggressive hepatitis	21	17	4(2+2[a,b,c])	—	7(5+2[b,c])	12	12	5(3+2[c])	15
(3) Less active cirrhosis	3	1	—	2[a,b,c]	—	1	—	1	1
(4) Active cirrhosis (20)[d]	18	13	1[a,b,c]	6(2+4[a,b,c])	5	10(9+1[b,c])	8	6(2+4[c])	10
Total	51	35	5	13	13	26	21	14	29
2. ACUTE HEPATITIS									
(1) Fully developed acute hepatitis	3	—	—	1	—	—	—	1	—
(2) Later and residual stages of acute hepatitis	3	—	—	2	—	—	—	—	—
Total	6	—	—	3	—	—	—	1	—
3. ACUTE HEPATITIS WITH SIGNS OF TRANSITION TO CHRONICITY	5	3	2[a,b,c]	—	1	2	2	1	3
4. NEAR NORMAL LIVER	4	—	—	4	—	—	—	—	—
TOTAL	66	38	7	20	14	28	23	16	32

a : HBcAg negative
b : negative for VCF
c : negative for Ig
d : 2 cases HBsAg tissue positive but serum negative

with CAH positive for both anti-HBs and anti-HBc was negative for IgG). In the 6 remaining VCF positive biopsies (Table 5.2) (CAH – 2: active cirrhosis – 4) no immunoglobulins were detected although a very small number of liver cell nuclei were positive for HBcAg and anti-HBc could be assayed in the blood.

In the cases of HBsAg positive acute hepatitis, no immunoglobulins were observed in the liver although they had anti-HBc in the blood. In AHTC. IgG could be visualized in all 3 VCF positive livers, and all had high titres of anti-HBc. None had anti-HBs in the blood. In HBsAg carriers ('near normal livers') there was no intrahepatic deposition of immunoglobulins despite presence of circulating anti-HBc.

The two patients with active cirrhosis with intrahepatic HBsAg and circulating anti-HBc, had no HBcAg, VCF nor IgG. HBcAg, VCF and immunoglobulins were not detected in cases of both acute and chronic hepatitis which were negative for HBsAg in the liver and serum, although some patients had anti-HBs and anti-HBc in the blood (Table 5.1).

The distribution of VCF and immunoglobulins in the hepatocytes of treated and non-treated patients appeared similar.

Discussion

The pathogenesis of liver cell damage in hepatitis B remains largely hypothetical. Theoretically, different immune mechanisms may be involved: humoral immunity to HBcAg or HBsAg, and cell-mediated immunity (be it antibody dependent or not) to HBsAg and HBcAg.

This immunofluorescence study confirms our previous finding of a strong correlation between membrane-localized HBsAg and the presence of HBcAg in aggressive forms of liver disease (CAH and active cirrhosis) characterized histologically by piecemeal necrosis and mononuclear cell infiltration.

The present study shows further correlation between the intrahepatic presence of HBcAg. VCF. immunoglobulins deposition and circulating anti-HBc in CAH. active cirrhosis and AHTC. This strong correlation among the above components is summarized in Figure 5.4. This relation also exists in CPH and less active cirrhosis where HBcAg is present in less though variable amounts. On the other hand in the majority of cases with acute hepatitis and in histologically near normal liver, no HBcAg was observed and, concomitantly, no VCF was demonstrated although all these patients had circulating anti-HBc. Moreover in acute exacerbation of CAH and active cirrhosis and in fully developed acute hepatitis, HBcAg was either absent or detected only in a very small number of cells: accordingly the number of VCF positive cells observed was relatively

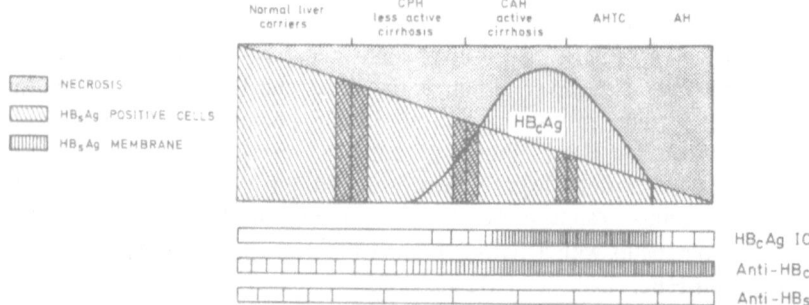

Figure 5.4 Shows strong correlation between hepatocytic membrane-localized HBsAg, HBcAg immune complexes and circulating anti-HBc but not with anti-HBs

low indicating a parallel relationship between HBcAg positivity and VCF capacity.

The demonstration of *in vitro* complement fixation in the livers of only HBsAg positive patients suggests the presence of immune complexes in the hepatocytes. The character and composition of these immune complexes are unclear. Most probably, they consist, not only in the nucleus but also in the cytoplasm, of HBcAg immune complexes rather than of HBs immune complexes, because of the following reasons:

(1) *In vitro* complement fixation was only observed in HBcAg positive biopsies, and irrespective of the types of liver morphology.
(2) All the cases positive for *in vitro* complement fixation had also circulating anti-HBc but only few had detectable anti-HBs in the blood.
(3) Elution studies performed by Ten Kate *et al.* (1974) and Gerber *et al.* (1976) identified the nuclear IgG as containing anti-HBc. In view of the recent demonstration of hepatitis B e antigen (HBeAg) in the hepatocytic nuclei by Arnold *et al.* (1977), the possibility may remain, however, that the nuclear IgG may also be of anti-HBe character and the eluate, in addition to anti-HBc, may contain anti-HBe or any other unknown antibodies. However, the rare presence of anti-HBe in the serum of HBeAg positive chronic hepatitis (Trepo *et al.*, 1976) may at least exclude the IgG as being anti-HBe.
(4) The double staining procedures performed with the application of contrast colour fluorochromes indicate that in VCF positive livers all cells expressing HBcAg also fix complement.

For unknown reasons, it was difficult to show IgG in the liver cell cytoplasm, but a high rate of detection of cytoplasmic *in vitro* complement fixation and even of cytoplasmic HBcAg was achieved. The intracytoplasmic distribution of complement fixation and of HBcAg were similar, while HBsAg was frequently found only in the hepatocytic membrane in the same biopsies. For all these reasons, it seems likely that the substrate for *in vitro* complement fixation, whether in the nucleus or in the cytoplasm, consists of HBcAg immune complexes.

The mechanisms of passage of immunoglobulin molecules into the hepatocytes are still obscure. Huang (1975) considered the possibility that this phenomenon might be an artefact, i.e. resulting from the influx of autologous anti-HBc during tissue processing. There is, however, no final proof that this phenomenon is indeed an artefact. Artificial displacement of IgG inside liver cells is even hard to conceive when, as in the present study, liver biopsies are immediately frozen. Furthermore, some biopsies in this study exhibited HBcAg in the nuclei without having demonstrable IgG and without fixing complement *in vitro*, although anti-HBc was positive in the blood. If nuclear IgG were an artefact of tissue preparation, there is no logical explanation for the lack of this 'artefact' in this group of cases submitted to strictly identical procedures of tissue preparation.

We therefore suggest that the presence of immunoglobulin in hepatocytes in hepatitis B virus infection is a genuine, *in vivo* phenomenon. Conceivably, the presence of HBsAg in the hepatocytic membranes (mostly in CAH and active cirrhosis), perhaps in conjuction with immune reactions at the level of the hepatocytic surface, may render the cells permeable to immunoglobulin, resulting in the entry and transport of immunoglobulin in the hepatocytes and leading to the formation of HBcAg immune complexes inside the cells.

In this view, neither the presence of HBcAg nor the presence of HBc antigen–antibody complexes can be held responsible for cell death, given the high frequency in chronic HB infection of cells which show either HBcAg or its complexes. Nevertheless, one might envisage a mechanism whereby these complexes lead to cytolysis, namely, when the complement system is also transported and activated in the cells. Cytolysis should be rapid in this case, since *in vivo* complement fixation has not been visualized. In this respect, humoral immune mechanisms related to HBcAg remain a possible mechanism for elimination of HBcAg containing hepatocytes.

The frequent finding of HBsAg in the hepatocytic membrane and cytoplasm of chronically infected liver – as well as its increased presence, together with an increased presence of HBcAg, in immunosuppressed patients with minimal liver damage (Ray *et al.*, 1976) – precludes that

HBsAg would be cytotoxic *per se*. In a previous report, based on the direct correlation between membrane-localized HBsAg and periportal piece-meal necrosis, we stressed the possible role of cell mediated immunity for the liver cell injury in chronic aggressive forms of hepatitis (Ray *et al.*, 1976). Available evidence suggests a role of cell mediated immune mechanisms related to HBsAg in eliminating HBsAg containing hepato-cytes (Dudley *et al.*, 1972; Ito *et al.*, 1972; Laiwah *et al.*, 1973).

Among the various possible immune mechanisms, the role of HBsAg immune complexes for the development of hepatitis B have been given least consideration because of the obvious difficulty of demonstrating circu-lating anti-HBs in the presence of HBsAg. However, HBsAg immune complexes have been found in the early stages of acute hepatitis B (Shulman and Barker, 1969; Almeida and Waterson, 1969) and anti-HBs, with the present methods, is detected in fulminant hepatitis B (Woolf *et al.*, 1976). In the presence of circulating HBsAg, HBsAg immune complexes have been shown in extrahepatic localizations in glomerulonephritis (Brzosko *et al.*, 1974), periateritis nodosa (Gocke *et al.*, 1970), and arth-ritis (Wands *et al.*, 1975). In these localizations, the complexes are seques-tered in special structures (e.g. glomerular basement membrane) where immune damage may be compatible with more prolonged cellular survival than in the HBsAg-producing hepatocyte. Thus present evidence indicates that humoral immune mechanisms in relation to HBsAg are rather involved in producing extrahepatic disease. Taking into account all the evidence available, it can be summarized that in the development of hepatitis B, there must be involvement of multiple immune mechanisms directed against HBV components which by themselves are non-injurious to the liver cell.

References

Almeida, J. D. and Waterson, D. P. (1969). Immune complexes in hepatitis. *Lancet*, 2, 983

Arnold, W., Nielsen, J. O., Hardt, F. and Meyer zum Buschenfelde, K. H. (1977). Localization of e-antigen in nuclei of hepatocytes in HBsAg-positive liver disease. *Gut*, 18, 994

Brzosko, W. J., Krawczynski, K., Nararewicz, T., Morzycka, M. and Nowoslawski, A. (1974). Glomerulonephritis associated with hepatitis B surface antigen immune complexes in children. *Lancet*, 2, 477

Burkholer, P. M. (1961). Complement fixation in diseases tissues: fixation of guinea pig complement in sections of kidney from humans with membranous glomerulonephritis and rats injected with anti-rat kidney serum. *J. Exp. Med.*, 114, 605

Dudley, F. J., Fox, R. A. and Sherlock, S. (1972). Cellular immunity and hepatitis associated Australian antigen in liver disease. *Lancet*, 1, 723

Gerber, M. A., Sarno, E. and Vernance, S. J. (1976). Immune complex in hepatocytic nuclei of HBAg positive chronic hepatitis. *N. Engl. J. Med.*, 294, 922

Gocke, D. J., Hsu, K., Morgan, C., Bombardieri, S., Lockshin, M. and Christain, C. L. (1970). Association between polyarteritis and Australia antigen. *Lancet*, **2**, 1149

Huang, S. (1975). Structural and immunoreactive characteristics of hepatitis B core antigen. *Am. J. Med. Sci.*, **270**, 131

Ito, K., Nakagawa, J. and Okimota, Y. (1972). Chronic hepatitis: migration inhibition of leucocytes in presence of Australia antigen. *N. Engl. J. Med.*, **286**, 1005

Laiwah, A. A. C. Y., Chaudhury, A. K. R. and Anderson, J. R. (1973). Lymphocyte transformation and leucocyte migration inhibition by Australia antigen. *Clin. Exp. Immunol.*, **15**, 27

Nowoslawski, A., Krawczynski, K., Brzosko, W. J. and Medalinski, K. (1972). Tissue localization of Australia antigen immune complex in acute and chronic hepatitis and liver cirrhosis. *Am. J. Path.*, **68**, 31

Ray, M. B., Desmet, V. J., Bradburne, A. F., Desmyter, J., Fevery, J. and De Groote, J. (1976). Differential distribution of hepatitis B surface antigen and hepatitis B core antigen in the liver of hepatitis B patients. *Gastroenterology*, **71**, 462

Ray, M. B., Desmet, V., Bradburne, A. F., Desmyter, J., Fevery, J. and De Groote, J. (1979). Hepatitis B core antigen immune complex in the liver of hepatitis B patients. *Clin. Exp. Immunol.* (In press)

Shulman, N. R. and Barker, L. F. (1969). Virus-like antigen, antibody and antigen–antibody complexes in hepatitis measured by complement fixation. *Science*, **165**, 304

Ten Kate, F. J. W., Feltkamp-Vroom, T., Helder, A. W., Roos, C. R. and van Blankenstein, M. (1974). Demonstration of HB antigens in liver tissue. *Digestion*, **10**, 305

Trepo, C. G., Magnius, L. O., Schaefer, R. A. and Prince, A. M. (1976). Detection of e antigen and antibody: correlations with hepatitis B surface and hepatitis B core antigens, liver disease and outcome in hepatitis B infections. *Gastroenterology*, **71**, 804

Wands, J. R., Alpert, E. and Isselbacher, K. J. (1975). Arthritis associated with chronic active hepatitis. *Gastroenterology*, **69**, 1256

Woolf, I. L., El Sheikh, N., Cullens, H., Lee, W. M., Eddleston, A. L. W. F., Williams, R. and Zuckerman, A. J. (1976). Enhanced HBsAg production in pathogenesis of fulminant viral hepatitis type B. *Br. Med. J.*, **2**, 669

6
Demonstration of hepatitis B surface antigen in the liver of patients with hepatocellular carcinoma

A possible link between HBV infection and hepatocellular carcinoma (HCC) was reported in 1970 (Sherlock *et al.*, 1970; Vogel *et al.*, 1970) but the full extent of the association was established only recently as more sensitive methods of detection of several markers of HBV infection in serum became available (Maupas *et al.*, 1975; Maupas *et al.*, 1977; Tabor *et al.*, 1977). This observation promoted the search for viral antigens in liver tissue to assess the oncogenic potential of HBV. In previous studies HBsAg was demonstrated in the non-cancerous part of the liver (Peters, 1975; Hadziyannis *et al.*, 1976). Recently the antigen has not only been observed in cancerous hepatocytes in the liver (Shikata, 1976; Nazarewicz *et al.*, 1977) but also in hepatoma metastisized in bone (Doury *et al.*, 1977).

The present study investigates the cellular localization patterns of HBsAg in 44 liver specimens with the histological diagnosis of HCC (Kew *et al.*, in preparation). HBsAg was demonstrated by immunofluorescence, PAP and orcein stain. This study also provides information regarding the relative sensitivity of the above techniques applied to large numbers of specimens.

Materials and methods

The present investigations were carried out on 44 liver specimens received from Dr M. C. Kew of Johannesbourg. The liver specimens were collected at autopsy from cases with the clinical diagnosis of liver cancer. Tissues were fixed in formalin and subsequently embedded in paraffin. Sections were mounted on glass slides and shipped to Leuven for examination.

Results

The 44 specimens were diagnosed histologically as HCC with or without cirrhosis. Twenty-eight of the 44 cases (64%) with HCC were associated with cirrhosis (Table 6.1); most of these (90%) were histologically less active.

Table 6.1 Incidence of cirrhosis and HBsAg in liver specimens with hepatocellular carcinoma

		HBsAg+	HBsAg−
HCC present			
(a) with cirrhosis	28	16	12
(b) without cirrhosis	16	3	13
Total	44	19 (43%)	25

Incidence in HBsAg in HCC

HBsAg was demonstrated in 13 (30%) specimens by all three procedures; an additional 6 were positive by both immunofluorescence and PAP methods. Therefore a total of 19 (43%) cases were positive for HBsAg. Of the 19 positive specimens, 16 had cirrhosis (84%), mostly of the macro-nodular type. No HBsAg was demonstrated in 25 liver specimens of which only 12 (48%) were cirrhotic. Therefore cirrhosis was more prevalent in HBsAg positive HCC than in the antigen negative group.

Table 6.2 shows the results obtained by immunohistochemistry and orcein stain. In HCC with cirrhosis, 10 had HBsAg in only the non-cancerous hepatocytes, 3 showed positivity exclusively in the cancerous tissue and 3 had HBsAg in both cancerous and non-cancerous areas. On the other hand in cases of HCC without cirrhosis 2 were positive in the cancerous cells, 1 in both areas, and none in the normal tissue only. Immunofluorescence and PAP gave identical positivity while no HBsAg was demonstrated in cancerous cells by the orcein stain (Table 6.2).

Table 6.2 Comparison of the results obtained by immunohistochemistry and by orcein stain

Histological diagnosis	Total positivity	IF			PAP			Orcein		
		Normal cell	Cancer cell	Both	Normal cell	Cancer cell	Both	Normal cell	Cancer cell	Both
HCC										
(a) cirrhosis	16	10	3	3	10	3	3	12	—	—
(b) without cirrhosis	3	—	2	1	—	2	1	1	—	—
Total	19	10	5	4	10	5	4	13	—	—

Localization patterns of HBsAg in HCC

HBsAg in the non-cancerous areas–In the cirrhotic nodules, the positive cells were frequently found in groups along the fibrous septa (Figure 6.1). The remaining area was either entirely negative or seeded with a few scattered positive cells. However, the number of HBsAg containing hepatocytes was remarkably low compared to that usually observed in liver biopsies from patients with less active cirrhosis (Ray *et al.*, 1976).

At the cellular level, HBsAg showed mostly a focal cytoplasmic distribution, a pattern which is commonly observed in patients with chronic hepatitis seronegative for HBsAg (Ray *et al.*, 1976). However, in the non-

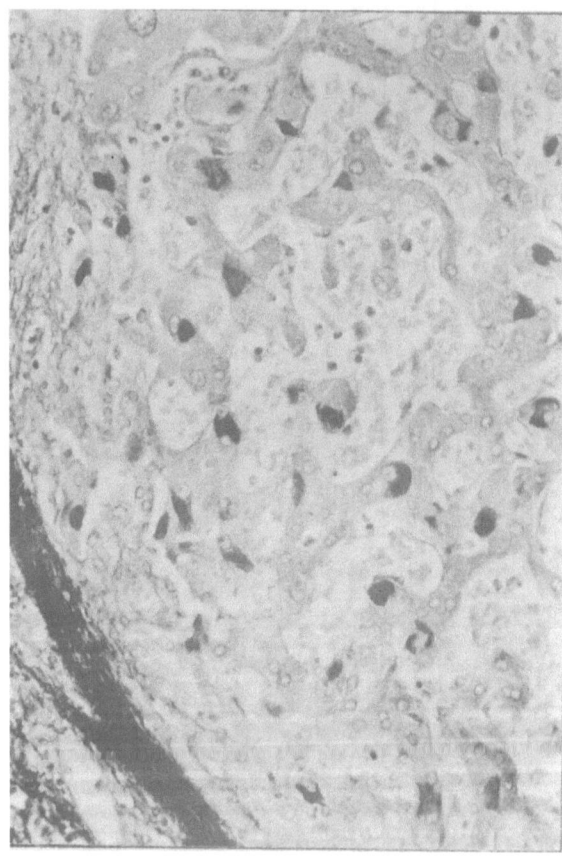

Figure 6.1 Hepatocellular carcinoma with cirrhosis: HBsAg is demonstrated focally in the cytoplasm of a group of hepatocytes present near the fibrous septa: PAP method (×210)

cancerous hepatocytes the antigen was observed frequently in a small focal area of the cytoplasm in contrast to the cancerous cells where it was usually located in the perinuclear area.

HBsAg in the cancerous areas. Although a total of 9 specimens showed HBsAg positivity in the tumour areas, the number of positive cells and the amount of antigen in the hepatoma cells were extremely low. A scanty amount of HBsAg was demonstrated only in the perinuclear area. Moreover, HBsAg was more readily detectable in moderately differentiated than in poorly differentiated HCC (Figure 6.2).

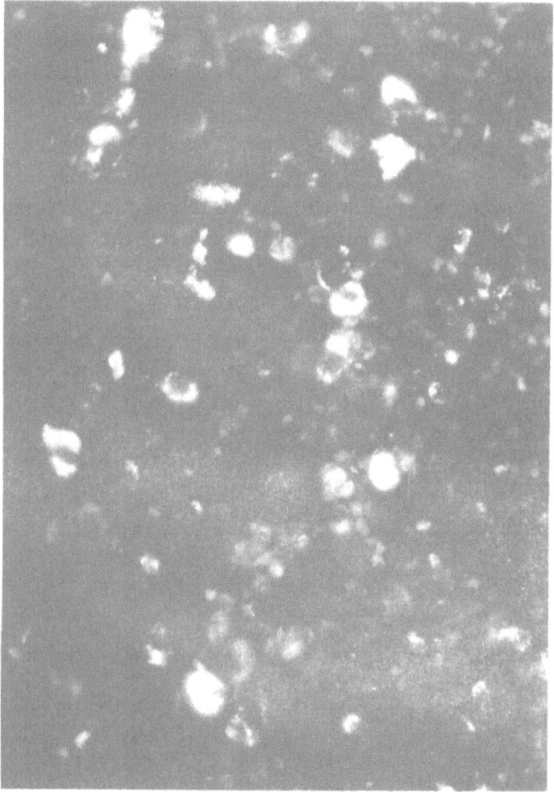

Figure 6.2 Hepatocellular carcinoma with cirrhosis. HBsAg is demonstrated in different cytoplasmic locations in few hepatoma cells. Indirect immunofluorescence (× 210)

Discussion

In the present study, HBsAg was demonstrated in paraffin embedded liver specimens by immunohistochemical methods (i.e. immunofluorescence and PAP procedures) and by orcein stain. Immunofluorescence and PAP techniques were found to be equally sensitive and gave identical results in each case. Orcein stain failed to detect HBsAg in the hepatoma cells and in one specimen in the non-cancerous tissue. These findings further confirm the previous observation that immunohistochemical methods are more sensitive than the orcein stain (Chapter 2).

HBsAg was demonstrated in the liver of 43% of cases with HCC. This frequency is slightly less than that reported for HBsAg in the serum as detected by RIA in a larger number of patients from the same country (MacNab et al., 1976). The observation that only very few cells are positive in a relatively large specimen again raises the problem of 'sampling error'. The figure of a 64% incidence of cirrhosis in HCC is very close to that reported by Kew et al.. (1974).

In the HBsAg positive HCC group 84% (16 of 19) had cirrhosis in contrast to only 48% in the antigen negative group. This finding enforces the previous contention that cirrhosis is a potentially precancerous condition and that HBV unquestionably is one of the aetiological factors in both cirrhosis and HCC. The incidence of HBsAg in HCC obtained in different parts of the world is summarized in Table 6.3.

The intrahepatic distribution of HBsAg in HCC is remarkable. The antigen is mostly observed in small focal areas of the hepatocytic cytoplasm (non-cancerous cells) or in the perinuclear area in hepatoma cells. This characteristic distribution pattern was previously observed in a study of

Table 6.3   Incidence of serum HBsAg in HCC patients in different countries

Country	Method*	HBsAg in HCC	HBsAg in Normal population	
Japan	IAHA	40%	3%	Nishioka (1973)
Taiwan	ID	80%	15%	Tong et al. (1971)
India	IEOP	64%	0.1%	Anand (1971)
South Africa	RIA	60%	9%	Kew et al. (1974)
Great Britain	RIA	24%	0.1%	Reed et al. (1973)
USA	RIA	26%	0.1%	Tabor et al. (1977)

*IAHA: Immune adherence haemagglutination
 ID: Ouchterlony immunodiffusion
 IEOP: Immunoelectrophoresis

the liver of chronic hepatitis patients seronegative for HBsAg having very low titres of HBsAg in the serum (Ray *et al.*, 1976). Therefore this focal intracytoplasmic distribution of HBsAg both in the cancerous and non-cancerous cells may suggest that the rate of antigen synthesis by the hepatocytes in HCC is lower than in cases with HBsAg positive chronic hepatitis. However, this assumption should be substantiated by estimating HBsAg titres in serial serum samples from patients with HCC and by comparing the results with those obtained in patients with chronic hepatitis B.

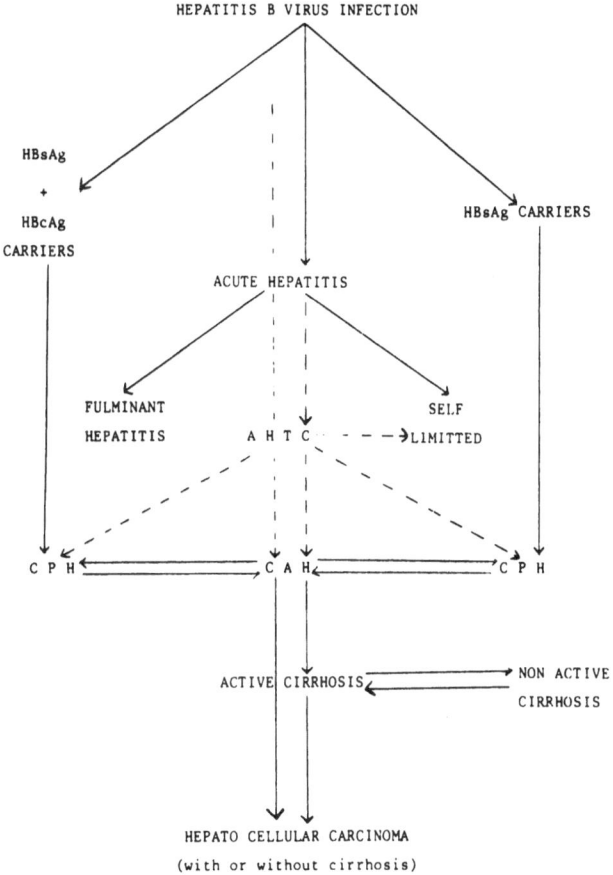

Figure 6.3 Schematic representation of natural histological evolution of HBV infection in the development of hepatocellular carcinoma. Broken lines indicate doubtful linkage although definite histological entities exist. As opposed to 'HBsAg Carriers', 'HBsAg + HBcAg Carriers' are extremely rare; their existence is only recently recognized; their immunopathological and serological status have yet to be determined

97

The amount of HBsAg in normal as compared with cancerous cells varied markedly: the highest amount of antigen was observed in normal hepatocytes, an intermediate amount in well differentiated hepatoma cells and very little or none in pleomorphic or anaplastic hepatoma cells. This phenomenon of a progressive decrease of cytoplasmic HBsAg may suggest that absence of HBsAg in the blood, liver or tumour does not exclude HBV as one of the aetiological factors in the development of HCC.

The oncogenic potential of HBV in the development of HCC is not known. It has been suggested that, at the beginning of the process, it is necessary for the viral genome to integrate in the host genome (Maupas et al., 1977). HBV is a small double stranded DNA virus and is reported to be a good candidate for integration (Hirschman, 1975). This phenomenon could block the production of viral proteins and switch on the synthesis of transplantation and tumour antigens (Allen and Cole, 1972). This may also explain the presence of only a small amount of HBsAg in the cancerous hepatocytes. The present study does not provide information regarding the demonstration of HBcAg in HCC. However, two recent studies (Maupas et al., 1977; Nazarewicz et al., 1977) reported absence of HBcAg in hepatoma cells.

Alternatively HBV itself may not be oncogenic but the long persistence of HBV antigens in the hepatocytes may create an ideal condition which promotes the carcinogenic potential of other environmental carcinogens. This hypothesis may explain the high prevalence of HCC in Africa and East Asia where biological hepatocarcinogens, e.g. aflatoxins, are fairly common. Figure 6.3 illustrates the hypothetical connection between HBV infection and hepatocellular carcinoma. Several other factors, such as genetic predisposition and hormonal factors, may also play an important role in the initiation and development of HCC.

References

Allen, D. W. and Cole, P. (1972). Viruses and human cancer. N. Engl. J. Med., 286, 70

Anand, S. (1971). Hepatitis associated antigen in primary liver cell carcinoma. Lancet, 2, 1032

Doury, J. C., Roche, J. C. and Brisou, B. (1977). Mise en évidence de l'AgHBs dans une métastase osseuse d'hepatome. Nouv. Presse Méd., 6, 2751

Hadziyannis, S., Giustozi, A., Moussouros, A. and Merikas, G. (1976). Hepatitis B core and surface antigens in the liver in primary liver cell carcinoma. In C. M. Leevy (ed.). Diseases of the Liver and Biliary Tract. pp. 174–178. (Basel: Karger)

Hirschman, S. Z. (1975). Integrator enzyme hypothesis for replication of hepatitis B virus. Lancet, 2, 436

Kew, M. C., Geddes, E. W., MacNab, G. M. and Bersohn, I. (1974). Hepatitis B antigen and cirrhosis in Bantu patients with primary liver cancer. Cancer, 34, 539

Kew, M. C., Ray, M. B. and Desmet, V. J. (in preparation)

MacNab, G. M., Urbanowicz, J. M., Geddes, E. W. and Kew, M. C. (1976). Hepatitis B surface antigen and antibody in Bantu patients with primary hepatocellular cancer. *Br. J. Canc.*, **33**, 544

Maupas, Ph., Werner, B. and London, W. T. (1975). Antibody to hepatitis B core antigen in patients with primary hepatic carcinoma. *Lancet*, **2**, 9

Maupas, Ph., Coursaget, P., Goudeau, A., Drucker, J., Sankale, M., Linhard, J. and Diebolt, G. (1977). Hepatitis B virus and primary liver carcinoma: evidences for a filiation hepatitis B, cirrhosis and primary liver cancer. *Ann. Microbiol. (Inst. Pasteur)*, **128**, 245

Nazarewicz, T., Krawczynski, K., Slusarczyk, J. and Nowoslawski, A. (1977). Cellular localization of hepatitis B virus antigens in patients with hepatocellular carcinoma co-existing with liver cirrhosis. *J. Infect. Dis.*, **135**, 298

Nishioka, K. (1973). Report of WHO associated workshop on hepatitis B antigen. (WHO)

Peters, R. L. (1975). Viral hepatitis: a pathological spectrum. *Am. J. Med. Sci.*, **270**, 17

Ray, M. B., Desmet, V. J., Fevery, J., De Groote, J., Bradburne, A. F. and Desmyter, J. (1976). Distribution patterns of hepatitis B surface antigen (HBsAg) in the liver of hepatitis patients. *J. Clin. Path.*, **29**, 94

Reed, W. D., Eddleston, A. L. W. F., Stern, R. B., Williams, R., Zuckerman, A. J., Bowes, A. and Earl, P. M. (1973). Detection of hepatitis B antigen by radioimmunoassay in chronic liver disease and hepatocellular carcinoma in Great Britain. *Lancet*, **2**, 690

Sherlock, S., Fox, R. A., Niazi, S. P. and Scheuer, P. J. (1970). Chronic liver disease and primary liver cell cancer with hepatitis-associated (Australia) antigen in serum. *Lancet*, **2**, 1243

Shikata, T. (1976). Primary liver carcinoma and liver cirrhosis. In K. Okuda, R. L. Peters (eds.). pp. 53–71. (J. Wiley and Sons)

Tabor, E., Gerety, R. J., Vogel, C. L., Bayley, A. C., Anthony, P. P., Chan, C. H. and Barker, L. F. (1977). Hepatitis B virus infection and primary hepatocellular carcinoma. *J. Natl. Canc. Inst.*, **58**, 1197

Tong, M. J., Sun, S. C., Schaeffer, B. T., Chang, N. K., Lo, K. J. and Peters, R. L. (1971). Hepatitis-associated antigen and hepatocellular carcinoma in Taiwan. *Ann. Intern. Med.*, **75**, 687

Vogel, C. L., Anthony, P. P., Mody, N. and Barker, L. F. (1970). Hepatitis-associated antigen in Ugandan patients with hepatocellular carcinoma. *Lancet*, **2**, 621

PART II
Experimental hepatitis and therapy

7
Development of hepatitis B in chimpanzees

Chimpanzees are considered to be the ideal non-human primates in which to study the development of hepatitis B (Maynard *et al.*, 1972; Desmyter *et al.*, 1973; Barker *et al.*, 1973; 1975) and the effectiveness of drugs (Desmyter *et al.*, 1976; Purcell *et al.*, 1976) and vaccines (Buynak *et al.*, 1976) for this disease.

The present study determines the infectivity of human serum containing HBsAg and investigates the pathogenetic processes involved during the development of hepatitis B by monitoring the appearance of HBV components in blood and liver. The histological and immunopathological alterations in the liver biopsies are correlated with the clinical symptoms and biochemical findings.

Materials and methods

Two adult male chimpanzees of 70 kg body weight (average) were the subjects of the present investigation. They were considered susceptible to HBV infection as their initial blood samples were repeatedly negative for HBsAg, anti-HBs and anti-HBc.

The animals were caged individually and fed with usual commercial diets. Blood counts and serum enzymes were determined before inoculation of chimp no. 1 (Mano) while chimp no. 2 (Dorus) served as control.

Inoculum

Serum from a HBsAg positive (subtype ayw) patient had been submitted to ultracentrifugation and the pellet examined by electron microscopy. The pellet revealed a heterogeneous population of Dane particles, 20 nm spheres and filamentous forms of HBsAg. The material was resuspended in 3 ml of tris-HCl buffer. 1.5 ml was injected intravenously and 1.5 ml into the liver itself.

Serology

Each blood sample was assayed for HBsAg, anti-HBs and anti-HBc, routine haematological values, transaminases and total bilirubin. Post inoculation blood samples were examined at 3-weekly intervals for the first two and a half months, after revelation of the first seropositivity in Mano, on average weekly (4–10 days) for the following three and a half months, fortnightly for the next month and once a month for the last two months. Blood from the control chimp (Dorus) was collected at a similar interval as for Mano during the first three months and monthly for the last six months.

Liver biopsy

Liver specimens were obtained after inoculation at suitable intervals based on clinical and serological developments. Adequate amounts of liver tissue were obtained on each occasion and were processed for routine histology and immunofluorescence.

Immunofluorescence

Serial cryostat sections from each biopsy were processed for the demonstration of HBsAg, HBcAg, VCF and various immunoglobulins.

Results

Mano, who received HBsAg-containing serum, developed hepatitis. The control animal did not show any signs of HBV infection; both serology and liver biopsy remained negative for HBV antigens throughout the study period.

Appearance of HBV components in the circulation and correlation with serum transaminases

Mano became seropositive for HBsAg, subtype ayw, 10 weeks (2.5 months) after inoculation (Figure 7.1) and the antigen remained detectable for a period of 4 weeks. Anti-HBs appeared 4 weeks after the disappearance of HBsAg in the blood and remained in the circulation 2 years after the study. The titres of anti-HBs fluctuated between 1:8 and 1:32. Anti-HBc

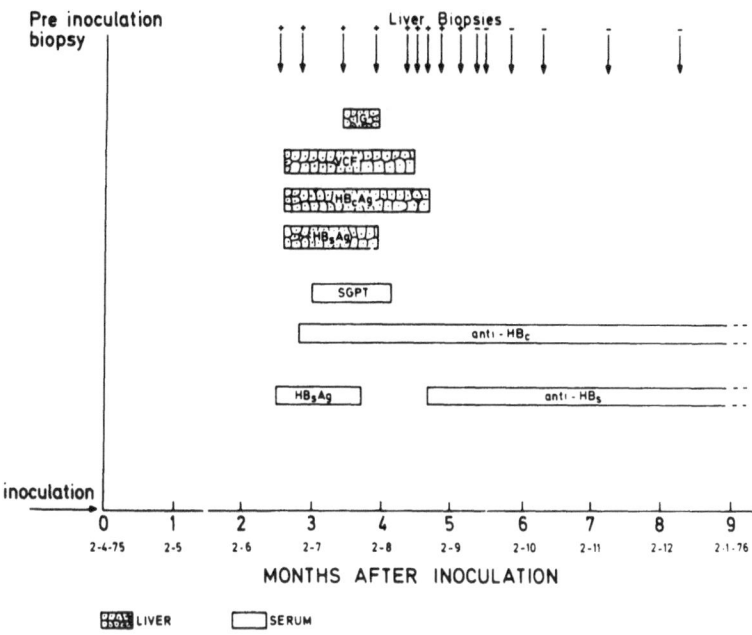

Figure 7.1   Course of HBV infection in Mano. Figure shows dynamics of serological and pathological changes after inoculation

was detectable 6 days after the appearance of HBsAg, became strongly positive after a week and remained detectable in low titres until at least 2 years after inoculation.

Serum transaminases (SGOT, SGPT, normal values below 30 IU/ml) rose suddenly with a peak value of 240 IU two weeks after HBsAg became positive – 8 days after the appearance of anti-HBc (Figure 7.1). Serum enzymes were abnormal for 6 weeks and became normal 2 weeks prior to the appearance of anti-HBs. However, serum transaminases sporadically became slightly abnormal until HBcAg was undetectable in the liver.

Bilirubin and other haematological values were within normal limits throughout the experiment.

Intrahepatic expression of HBV antigens, VCF and immunoglobulins: correlation with liver histology

Liver biopsy samples taken before the inoculation were negative for HBV antigens, VCF and immunoglobulin deposition. Positive immunofluorescence for HBV components was first observed in biopsy no. 2 taken 5 days after the serum became positive for HBsAg (i.e. 11 weeks after inoculation) (Table 7.1); HBsAg was demonstrated in the cell membranes but not in the cytoplasm in 25% of the hepatocytes. The fluorescence was moderate in intensity. HBcAg was localized only in the nuclei and rarely in the cytoplasm, its fluorescence was coarsely granular with a moderate to strong intensity. No immunoglobulin deposition was noted. At this time, liver histology was practically normal except for the presence of a very few small foci of lymphocytes in the lobular parenchyma apparently around individual necrotic hepatocytes. No portal infiltration was present.

Table 7.1 Intrahepatic distribution of HBV components, VCF and IgG in Mano

Biopsies	Date	HBsAg	HBcAg	VCF	IgG
1 (Inoculation)	02.04.75	—	—	—	—
2	21.06.75	+(25%)	+(30%)	+(30–40%)	—
3	30.06.75	++(60–80%)	++(55–65%)	++(50%)	—
4	17.07.75	+(60–70%)	++(55–60%)	++(50%)	+(10%)
5	31.07.75	+(5%)	+(1%)	+(10%)	+(0.1%)
6	14.08.75	—	+(0.1%)	+(5%)	—
7	19.08.75	—	±(0–1%)	+(1%)	—
8	25.08.75	—	±(0–0.1%)	—	—
9	01.09.75	—	—	—	—
10	08.09.75	—	—	—	—
11	15.09.75	——	—	—	—
12	19.09.75	—	—	—	—
13	30.09.75	—	—	—	—
14	13.10.75	—	—	—	—
15	10.11.75	—	—	—	—
16	10.12.75	—	—	—	—

In parentheses: approximate percentage of affected liver cells

In the following two biopsies (no. 3 and no. 4) collected approximately 13 and 15 weeks after the inoculation, HBsAg was demonstrated in the cell membranes of 60 to 80% of the hepatocytes (Figure 7.2). The fluorescence was strong and granular in character; a few Kupffer cells were also positive. HBcAg, VCF and IgG were demonstrated in the nuclei of approximately 60%, 50% and 10% of the cells respectively. Rarely VCF was observed in the hepatocytic cytoplasm. The liver biopsy no. 3 collected 13 weeks after inoculation showed signs of a slight hepatitis. There was slight to moderate mononuclear cell infiltration in the portal fields and sinusoidal spaces. Except for the presence of a few acidophilic bodies, there were no striking parenchymal changes. A liver biopsy obtained 15 weeks (no. 4) after inoculation showed features of mild acute hepatitis. Moderate to dense mononuclear cell infiltration with little 'spillover' was

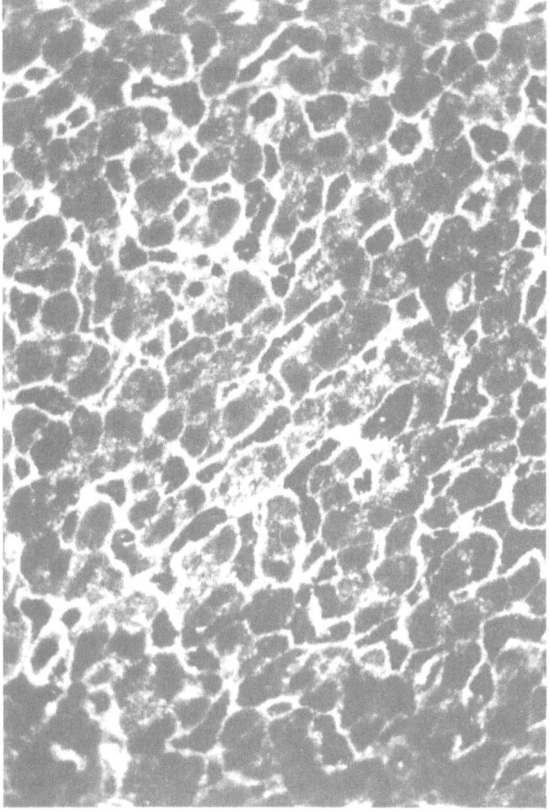

Figure 7.2 Liver biopsy no. 3: membrane-localized HBsAg is present in high numbers of hepatocytes; corresponding paraffin specimen showed slight hepatitis (× 230)

observed in most of the portal tracts (Figure 7.3). Acidophilic bodies were quite numerous and often found to be surrounded by mononuclear cells. The hepatocytes around a couple of centrilobular areas showed small foci of focal confluent necrosis which was mostly of the coagulative type. There was also accumulation of mononuclear cells in the centrilobular areas. Virtually no PAS positive pigmented macrophages were observed.

The next biopsy (no. 5), which was also the last specimen positive for HBsAg, collected 17 weeks after inoculation, showed faint to moderate fluorescence in the cell membranes of only about 5% of the hepatocytes. Faint to moderate HBcAg positivity was observed in only about 1% of the nuclei; however, 10% of the hepatocytic nuclei were positive for VCF, and IgG was demonstrated rarely (+ 0.1%). Liver histology showed

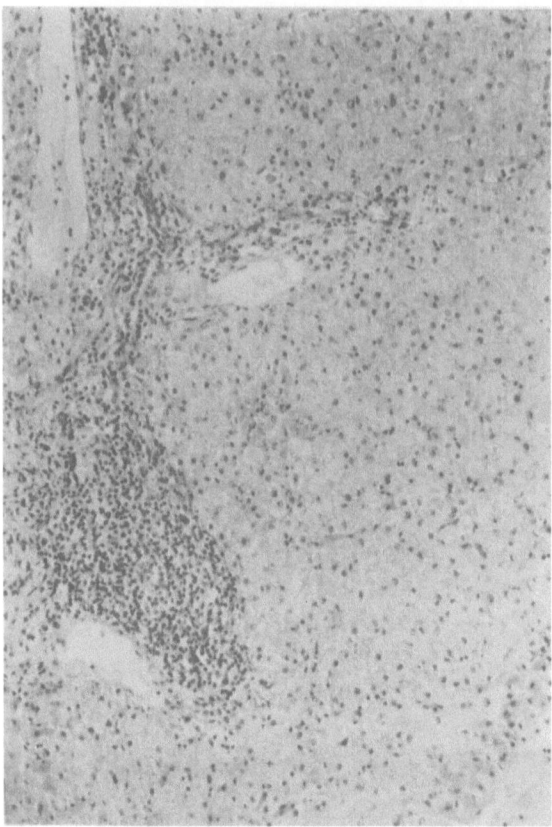

Figure 7.3 Routine histology: biopsy no. 4: picture of acute hepatitis. Moderate to dense mononuclear cell infiltration in the portal tract – no true 'piecemeal necrosis' is present (× 125)

a picture of non-specific reactive hepatitis. There was slight to moderate mononuclear cell infiltration in the portal tracts and sinusoids, a few acidophilic bodies and an occasional PAS positive pigmented macrophage was found.

All the subsequent liver specimens were negative for HBsAg. However, very few nuclei were still positive for HBcAg in three successive biopsies (nos. 6, 7 and 8). The last HBcAg positive biopsy was taken approximately 20 weeks after inoculation. In those liver specimens VCF was observed infrequently and no IgG was present. These three biopsies showed non-specific reactive hepatitis. Liver histology became normal at 24 weeks (five and a half months) after inoculation. All liver biopsies of the control chimpanzee remained unchanged.

Discussion

The present study reports the successful induction of hepatitis B in a chimpanzee by injecting HBsAg positive serum containing Dane particles. This further substantiates the previous contention that the Dane particle represents the aetiological agent of hepatitis B. Although viral hepatitis may occur spontaneously in chimpanzees (Desmyter *et al.*, 1971; Maynard *et al.*, 1971; Desmyter *et al.*, 1973), such development seems unlikely in the present case because of the appearance in the blood of the ayw subtype, identical to that of the inoculated serum. Moreover, the chronological sequence of the appearance of HBsAg in the blood and the biochemical evidence of hepatocellular injury as well as the demonstration of HBs and HBc antigens in the liver along with the histopathological changes indicate development of hepatitis B due to the inoculation. The present study confirms similar investigations done previously by Maynard *et al.* (1971) and Barker *et al.* (1973). The chimp did not develop hyperbilirubinaemia or any overt signs of clinical hepatitis. Signs of hepatocellular necrosis without icterus were also observed by Maynard *et al.* (1971) and are commonly encountered in anicteric hepatitis in man.

The observed sequence in the appearance of circulating HBsAg, anti-HBs and anti-HBc is classical in experimental hepatitis (Barker *et al.*, 1975; Hoofnagle *et al.*, 1975). Anti-HBs (1/32 PHA) appeared 4 weeks after the disappearance of HBsAg from the blood and remained detectable thereafter. Anti-HBc appeared earlier than anti-HBs in the presence of HBsAg. At the beginning anti-HBc titres were low but gradually increased and remained high throughout the experimental period, long after the disappearance of HBcAg from the liver.

Serum transaminases were elevated 9 days after the appearance of circulating anti-HBc and the appearance of HBcAg in the liver. Enzyme levels returned to normal approximately three weeks before the appearance of anti-HBs. Therefore, the HBcAg system appears to be more closely associated with hepatocellular necrosis than the HBsAg system.

HBcAg was observed in a few cells in the biopsy (no. 2) taken just after the serum became positive for HBsAg. However, the proportion of positive nuclei increased in the subsequent biopsies (nos. 3 and 4) taken at the height of hepatocellular damage. These findings also correlated with the presence of VCF and IgG deposition in the hepatocytic nuclei. The identification and significance of HBcAg immune complexes in the hepatocytes of HBcAg positive chronic hepatitis were discussed in Chapter 5.

The possibility that HBsAg immune complexes caused hepatocytic damage is considered less likely as anti-HBsAg was only detectable after subsidence of the disease. However, the expression of HBsAg in the hepatocytic membranes at the early stage may render the cells susceptible for immune attack probably by T lymphocytes resulting in cell necrosis and mononuclear cell infiltration in the lobules and in the portal tracts. This hypothesis has been discussed in Chapter 3 and Chapter 4.

An interesting phenomenon is the demonstration of HBsAg, HBcAg and VCF in the liver specimens well after the disappearance of HBsAg from the circulation. HBsAg was demonstrable in the liver 15 days after its disappearance from the serum and HBcAg and VCF were still demonstrable even after one month. These observations are in contrast to the findings of Berquist et al. (1975) who reported the disappearance of hepatic HBcAg before HBsAg. However, the present findings confirm our previous observation (Ray et al., 1976) in human liver where HBsAg was more readily detected in the liver by immunofluorescence than in the serum by RIA. It has indeed been reported that RIA, although the most sensitive assay available, cannot detect HBsAg below the level of 10^{10} particles per ml of serum (Tabor et al., 1977).

The observed histological changes in the liver are comparable with features of acute hepatitis in man. Although there were significant amounts of mononuclear cell infiltration in the portal fields, typical piecemeal necrosis was not observed. The animal did not develop chronic hepatitis. Liver histology returned to normal five and a half months after inoculation (one month after HBcAg became negative in the tissue). Similar observations were made in chimpanzees by Barker and co-workers (1973) and in man by Hoofnagle et al. (1975). The exact cause for the development of chronicity is not known but it has been well established that different individuals react diversily after challenge with HBV (Hoofnagle et al., 1975).

References

Barker, L. F., Chisari, F. V., McGrath, P. P., Dalgard, D. W., Kirschstein, R. L., Almeida, J. D., Edgington, T. S., Sharp, G. D. and Peterson, M. R. (1973). Transmission of type B viral hepatitis to chimpanzees. *J. Infect. Dis.*, **127**, 648

Barker, L. F., Maynard, J. E., Purcell, R. H., Hoofnagle, J. L., Berquist, K. R. and London, W. T. (1975). Viral hepatitis type B in experimental animals. *Am. J. Med. Sci.*, **270**, 189

Berquist, K. R., Peterson, J. M., Murphy, B. L., Ebert, J. W., Maynard, J. E. and Purcell, R. H. (1975). Hepatitis B antigens in serum and liver of chimpanzees acutely infected with hepatitis B virus. *Infect. Immun.*, **12**, 602

Buynak, E. B., Roehm, R. R., Tytell, A. A., Bertland, A. U., Lampson, G. P. and Hilleman, M. R. (1976). Development and chimpanzee testing of a vaccine against human hepatitis B. *Proc. Soc. Exp. Biol. Med.*, **151**, 694

Desmyter, J., Liu, W., De Somer, P. and Mortelmans, J. (1971). Epidemic clustering of anti-HAA (Australia) antibodies in chimpanzees. *Bacteriol. Proc.*, 168

Desmyter, J., Liu, W. T., De Somer, P. and Mortelmans, J. (1973). Primates as the model for human viral hepatitis: transmission of infection by human hepatitis B virus. *Vox Sang. (Suppl.)*, **24**, 17

Desmyter, J., Ray, M. B., De Groote, J., Bradburne, A. F., Desmet, V. J., Edy, V. G., Billiau, A., De Somer, P. and Mortelmans, J. (1976). Administration of human fibroblast interferon in chronic hepatitis B infection. *Lancet*, **2**, 645

Hoofnagle, J. H., Gerety, R. J. and Barker, L. F. (1975). Antibody to hepatitis B core antigen. *Am. J. Med. Sci.*, **270**, 179

Maynard, J. E., Hartwell, W. V. and Berquist, K. R. (1971). Hepatitis-associated antigen in chimpanzees. *J. Infect. Dis.*, **123**, 660

Maynard, J. E., Berquist, K. R. and Krushak, D. H. (1972). Experimental infection of chimpanzee with the virus of hepatitis B. *Nature*, **237**, 514

Purcell, R. H., London, W. T., McAuliffe, V. J., Palmer, A. E., Kaplan, P. M., Gerin, J. L., Wagner, J., Popper, H., Lvovsky, E., Wong, D. C. and Levy, H. B. (1976). Modification of chronic hepatitis B virus infection in chimpanzees by administration of an interferon inducer. *Lancet*, **2**, 757

Ray, M. B., Desmet, V. J., Fevery, J., De Groote, J., Bradburne, A. F. and Desmyter, J. (1976). Hepatitis B surface antigen (HBsAg) in the liver of patients with hepatitis: a comparison with serological detection. *J. Clin. Path.*, **29**, 89

Tabor, E., Gerety, R. J., Vogel, C. L., Bayley, A. C., Anthony, P. P., Chan, C. H. and Barker, L. F. (1977). Hepatitis B virus infection and primary hepatocellular carcinoma. *J. Natl. Cancer Inst.*, **58**, 1197

8
Effect of human fibroblast interferon in chronic hepatitis B infection

At present there is no satisfactory treatment for chronic hepatitis B. Essentially the therapy is based upon the suppression of the immune system by corticosteroids and antimetabolites (Soloway *et al.*, 1972; Murray-Lyon *et al.*, 1973). However, such therapy may promote intrahepatic accumulation of viral antigen (Gudat, *et al.*, 1975; Ray *et al.*, 1976) and prolong the infection.

Therefore an alternative therapeutic agent is preferable. Interferon, an antiviral glycoprotein produced by many somatic cells during the replication of most RNA and DNA viruses (Carter and De Clerq, 1974) may be justified since it was found to be effective in the treatment of several other human viral infections (Merigan *et al.*, 1975). Moreover interferon does not cause obvious toxicity (Strander *et al.*, 1973; Jordan *et al.*, 1974). On the other hand interferon has not been detected in hepatitis B (Taylor and Zuckerman *et al.*, 1968; Wheelock *et al.*, 1968), suggesting that HBV is a poor inducer of interferon and that passive administration will not be redundant to endogenous interferon.

This study evaluates the therapeutic potency of human fibroblast interferon in chronic hepatitis B in man and in chimpanzees.

Materials and methods

Preparation of interferon

Interferon was prepared in human diploid fibroblasts, using double stranded RNA, Poly (I), Poly (c) and superinduction (Billiau *et al.*, 1973). It was purified and concentrated by fractional precipitation with ammonium sulphate, titrated by inhibition of replication of vesicular stomatitis virus in human diploid cells, using a dye uptake method (Finter, 1969), and calibrated against the Medical Research Council 69/19 standard of human interferon. Each dose contained 10^7 IU of human interferon in 10 ml volume. One treatment course consisted of seven doses injected intramuscularly on every alternate day.*

Subjects

Chimpanzees–Two male chimpanzees, weighing 60 kg each, had been chronic carriers of HBsAg since they were first examined. Their liver function tests and liver histology were in the normal range in the previous year. Liver biopsies were taken during general anaesthesia, 3 biopsies in three months before, one immediately before, 3 during treatment and 12 up to 4 months after treatment with interferon.

Patient–The patient, a 42-year-old male weighing 54 kg, had HBsAg positive CAH first diagnosed in 1969. He was given immunosuppressive drugs (cortison and azathioprine) two years before the treatment with interferon. No evaluation was noted in the year before interferon treatment. Serum SGOT and SGPT were abnormal and fluctuated between 30 and 100 IU/litre. The serum bilirubin level was consistently normal. A total of three liver biopsies was obtained, one immediately before, one immediately after and the last biopsy five weeks after the initiation of interferon treatment. Liver biopsies were processed for routine diagnosis, and immunofluorescent examinations.

Serology

Serum samples were collected at the time of each biopsy and assayed for HBV components. HBeAg antigen was determined by double immuno-diffusion (Magnius and Espmark, 1972).

Immunofluorescence

HBsAg and HBcAg were demonstrated in frozen liver specimens by immunofluorescence. The number of positive cells was expressed in approximate percentage.

---

*Interferon was prepared in the Laboratory of Professor P. De Somer, Rector K. U. Leuven, Rega Institute for Medical Research, Leuven, Belgium.

Results

Side effects of interferon

The treatment was first given to two chimpanzees and later on to the patient. None of them had demonstrable interferon in the blood before treatment. Injections of interferon were well tolerated and clinical, bio-chemical and haematological examinations showed no side effects. However, the patient had a rise of temperature up to 38 °C and was treated with aspirin. The temperature was not measured in the chimpanzees who required general anaesthesia for handling.

Changes in circulating and intrahepatic HBV components in chimpanzees

No change of serum titres of HBsAg was noted before and after treatment. They had no demonstrable anti-HBs. Immunofluorescence on all liver speci-mens showed weak peripheral cytoplasmic and membrane staining for HBsAg in 15% of the hepatocytes in both chimpanzees; this was not modified during or after treatment, the only exception was in chimpanzee 1, whose liver showed areas of full cytoplasmic positivity for HBsAg one to two weeks after treatment, and membrane expression was minimal at that time.

The most striking changes were seen in the HBc system. In chimpanzee 1, 15% of the hepatocytic nuclei stained positively for HBcAg in the pre-treatment biopsy. After one week of treatment, the number of positive nuclei and the intensity of staining decreased progressively during the sub-sequent five weeks when less than 0.5% of the nuclei were positive. The number of positive nuclei rose rapidly again and reached 30% after one month. Serum anti-HBc rose from a stable titre of 16 before and during treatment to 128 one week afterwards; this was maintained for six weeks and then declined. Chimpanzee 2 had no demonstrable HBcAg in the liver at any time. He had constant, high anti-HBc titres of 20000 before treatment; the anti-HBc titre fell to 128 after one week's treatment and remained at that level during the following weeks.

Changes in circulating and intrahepatic HBV components in patients

Table 8.1 summarizes the results obtained in the patients. The titres of HBsAg and anti-HBs (which was demonstrable only by RIA) did not change. However, a change was observed in HBsAg expression in the liver. The pretreatment biopsy specimen showed strong membrane-localized HBsAg in 90% of the cells and cytoplasmic staining in 5%. Immediately

Table 8.1 Effect of interferon on intrahepatic and serum HBV components in patient

	Pretreatment biopsy	Biopsy during treatment	Biopsy 5 wks after treatment
HBsAg	Membrane – 90% Cytoplasmic 5%	Membrane – 60% Cytoplasmic 15%	Membrane – 60% Cytoplasmic 35%
HBcAg	Nuclei – 30% Cytoplasmic ±	Nuclei – 20% Cytoplasmic –	Nuclei – 3% Cytoplasmic –
Anti-HBs	No change	No change	No change
Anti-HBc	No change	No change	No change

after treatment, there was membrane staining in 60% and cytoplasmic staining in 15% of the hepatocytes, both of moderate intensity. In the last biopsy specimen taken 5 weeks later, there was 60% membrane staining and 35% cytoplasmic staining, both of moderate intensity.

Changes were also observed in the HBcAg system. HBcAg was localized in 30% of the nuclei before treatment. Immediately after treatment 20% of the nuclei were positive at low intensity. Only 3% positive nuclei were observed five weeks after interferon administration. A few hepatocytes showed cytoplasmic HBcAg in the pretreatment biopsy specimens but not later. The serum anti-HBc titre of 3200 remained unchanged during the observation period.

The HBeAg antigen was not detectable in the serum of the patient or of the chimpanzees at any time of the study. Dane particles were rarely observed in sporadic serum samples from chimp 1 and the patient. These were absent in chimp 2.

No histological changes were observed in the liver biopsies from both chimpanzees and from the patient.

Shifts in intrahepatic HBV components are interferon specific

Evidence that the changes were due to treatment and not to unrelated spontaneous fluctuations in the expression of HBV antigens was as follows. No changes in HBV components were observed in the serial biopsy specimens taken from each chimp before treatment. The changes were observed only after interferon and were interpretable in terms of antiviral action. Moreover in 4 control patients, 3 with CAH with both HBsAg and HBcAg in the liver, and one apparently normal antigen carrier, with only HBsAg in the liver but no HBcAg, repeat biopsies were taken over a period of 2 years during which their histological and clinical status did not change; there were no changes in intrahepatic distribution of HBsAg and HBcAg. In contrast, five other HBsAg positive chronic hepatitis patients whose histological and clinical status did change also showed changing patterns of viral antigen in their livers.

Discussion

The results show that HBV infection is sensitive to interferon and that it is the HBcAg or nucleocapsid system which is primarily responsive. Reduction in HBcAg was seen after treatment in both livers with demonstrable HBcAg. Changes were also observed in the titres of circulating anti-HBc but were unrelated to intrahepatic HBcAg expressions. The titres of serum HBsAg were not modified but a shift from membrane staining to cytoplasmic staining was noted for HBsAg in the livers of two subjects. It is important to mention that in chronic hepatitis in man, predominant membrane staining for HBsAg is the hallmark of the aggressive form of the disease and coincides with a high level of nuclear HBcAg, while predominant cytoplasmic staining for HBsAg is the hallmark of clinically subdued, persistent forms and coincides with little or no demonstrable nuclear HBcAg (Chapter 2 and Chapter 3). Therefore interferon seems to have modified the expression of HBV antigens into a pattern associated with lower disease activity.

The changes in viral expression both in the blood and livers appeared to be short lived, at least in chimpanzees, although this needs further confirmation by additional observations. With other viruses, interferon treatment has not led to the eradication of the viral genome from cells with established chronic infection. Therefore it is well possible that the effects observed in this study could be annulled after withdrawal of the therapy. However, more prolonged treatment might have a longer effect by cell population dynamics – and eventually improve liver function and histology. This might be achieved by replacement of infected cells by uninfected cells which are protected against infection by interferon.

The present study reports the action of interferon in chronic hepatitis B, but this may be useful also in acute hepatitis B, since acute infection by other viruses is generally more readily influenced than chronic infection. Viruses which in acute infection are sensitive to interferon have been found to be both insensitive (Desmyter *et al.*, 1967) and sensitive (Billiau *et al.*, 1973) to interferon in chronic infection.

Since this study was published (Desmyter *et al.*, 1976), Greenberg *et al.* (1976) have reported that human leukocyte interferon depressed the HBcAg system in the blood of 3 patients with CAH; their livers were not examined. No change was noted in the HBsAg system. Shortly afterwards, Purcell *et al.* (1976) reported similar findings using an interferon inducer in chronically infected chimpanzees. The changes closely resembled those obtained with exogenous interferon. There was depression of HBcAg in the liver and DNA polymerase and HBeAg antigen levels fell sharply within 10 days of administration of the inducer. However, the action of the inducer, like that of fibroblast and leukocyte interferon, was short lived. These three studies are complementary to each other and agree in one point: that it is the HBcAg system which is depressed after using different agents with basically the same therapeutic effect; therefore the probable action of other substances suspected in unpurified interferon can be excluded.

The mechanism of action of interferon on hepatitis B is unknown. Greenberg *et al.* (1976) suggested that interferon may have acted via the immune system. But the action of the interferon on the immune system is still controversial: interferon has been found to be an immunological depressant rather than a stimulant (Demayer, 1976), while other studies reported it as a stimulant of both humoral and cellular immunity (Skurkovich *et al.*, 1973).

The present study represents the first application of human fibroblast interferon to man. Fibroblast interferon has the advantage over leukocyte interferon in that it can be produced in large quantities from easily growing cell lines – fibroblasts. Moreover, human fibroblast interferon is well tolerated, except for a febrile reaction which was also observed by others with leukocyte interferon.

References

Billiau, A., Joniau, M. and De Somer, P. (1973). Mass production of human interferon in diploid cells stimulated by Poly 1: c. *J. Gen. Virol.*, **19**, 1

Billiau, A., Sobis, H. and De Somer, P. (1973). Influence of interferon on virus particle formation in different oncornavirus carrier cell lines. *Int. J. Cancer*, **12**, 646

Carter, W. A. and De Clercq, E. (1974). Viral infection and host defense. *Science*, **186**, 1172

Demayer, E. (1976). Interferon and delayed-type hypersensitivity to a viral antigen. *J. Infect. Dis.*, **133**, A63

Desmyter, J., Rawls, W. E., Melnick, J. L., Yow, M. D. and Barrett, F. (1967). Interferon in congenital rubella: response to live attenuated measles vaccine. *J. Immunol.*, **99**, 771

Desmyter, J., Ray, M. B., De Groote, J., Bradburne, A. F., Desmet, V. J., Edy, V. G., Billiau, A., De Somer, P. and Mortelmans, J. (1976). Administration of human fibroblast interferon in chronic hepatitis B infection. *Lancet*, **2**, 645

Finter, N. B. (1969). Dye uptake methods for assessing viral cytopathogenicity and their application to interferon assays. *J. Gen. Virol.*, **5**, 419

Greenberg, H. B., Pollard, R. B., Lutwick, L. I., Gregory, P. B., Robinson, W. S. and Merigan, T. C. (1976). Effect of human leukocyte interferon on hepatitis B virus infection in patients with chronic active hepatitis. *N. Engl. J. Med.*, **295**, 517

Gudat, F., Bianchi, L., Sonnabend, W., Thiel, G., Aenishaenslin, W. and Stalder, G. A. (1975). Pattern of core and surface expression in liver tissue reflects state of specific immune response in hepatitis. *Lab. Invest.*, **32**, 1

HUMAN FIBROBLAST INTERFERON IN HEPATITIS B

Jordan, G. W., Fried, R. P. and Merigan, T. C. (1974). Administration of human leukocyte interferon in herpes zoster. 1. Safety, circulating anti-viral activity, and host responses to infection. *J. Infect. Dis.*, **130**, 56

Magnius, L. O. and Espmark, J. A. (1972). New specificities in Australia antigen positive sera distinct from the 'le Bouvier' determinants. *J. Immunol.*, **109**, 1017

Merigan, T. C., Jordan, G. W. and Fried, R. P. (1975). Clinical utilization of exogenous human interferon, anti-viral mechanisms. In M. Pollard (ed.). *Perspectives in Virology*, vol. 9. pp. 249–264. (New York: Academic Press)

Murray-Lyon, I. M., Stern, R. B. and Williams, R. (1973). Controlled trial of prednisone and azathioprine in active chronic hepatitis. *Lancet*, **1**, 735

Purcell, R. H., Gerin, J. L., London, W. T., Wagner, J., MCauliffe, V. J., Popper, H., Palmer, A. E., Lvovsky, E., Kaplan, P. M., Wong, D. C. and Levy, H. B. (1976). Modification of chronic hepatitis B virus infection in chimpanzees by administration of an interferon inducer. *Lancet*, **2**, 757

Ray, M. B., Desmet, V. J., Fevery, J., De Groote, J., Bradburne, A. F. and Desmyter, J. (1976). Differential distribution of hepatitis B surface antigen and hepatitis B core antigen in the liver of hepatitis B patients. *Gastroenterology*, **71**, 462

Skurkovich, S. V., Klinova, E. G., Aleksandrovskaya, I. M., Lavina, N. V., Arkhipovana and Bulicheva, T. I. (1973). Stimulation of transplantation immunity and plasma cell reaction by interferon in mice. *Immunology*, **25**, 317

Soloway, R. D., Summerskill, W. H. J., Baggenstoss, A. H., Geall, M. G., Gitnick, G. L., Elveback, I. R. and Schoenfield, L. J. (1972). Clinical, biochemical and histological remission of severe chronic active liver disease: a controlled study of treatments and early prognosis. *Gastroenterology*, **63**, 820

Strander, H., Cantell, K., Carlstrom, G. and Jakobsson, P. A. (1973). Clinical and laboratory investigations on man: systemic adminstration of potent interferon to man. *J. Natl. Cancer Inst.*, **51**, 733

Taylor, P. E. and Zuckerman, A. J. (1968). Non-production of interfering substances by serum from patients with infectious hepatitis. *J. Med. Microbiol.*, **1**, 217

Wheelock, E. F., Schenker, S. and Combes, B. (1968). Absence of circulating interferon in patients with infectious and serum heaptitis. *Proc. Soc. Exp. Biol. Med.*, **128**, 251

PART III
Demonstration of hepatitis B surface antigen in extrahepatic locations

9
Demonstration of hepatitis B surface antigen in the kidney of patients with glomerulonephritis

The co-existence of liver cirrhosis and glomerulonephritis was recognized nearly thirty years ago (Baxter and Ashworth *et al.*, 1946; Patek *et al.*, 1951). However, a common causative agent for both diseases entities could not be established immediately. Recently HBsAg was demonstrated both in the kidney and liver of patients with circulating HBsAg (Combes *et al.*, 1971; Knieser *et al.*, 1974) and focal glomerulonephritis has been produced in baboons (Gyorkey *et al.*, 1975) after inoculation with HBsAg containing plasma. These findings suggest that HBV may play a significant role in the pathogenesis of renal as well as hepatic disease. The present study investigates the prevalence of HBsAg in patients with glomerulonephritis and the detection of concomitant liver disease among those patients.

Materials and methods

Sixty-six kidney specimens obtained from 66 patients were included in this study. The patients were 16 to 65 years old; 75% were male. Some of the biopsies studied were from patients undergoing haemodialysis. As several biopsies were sent in from other hospitals, the exact number of haemodialysis patients was not available at the time of writing.

Immunofluorescence and serology

Serial cryostat sections from each biopsy were examined for HBsAg, immunoglobulins and complement B_1A/B_1C (C3).

Histological and immunofluorescence findings were used to classify the kidney specimens according to the criteria of Habib and Kleinknecht

(1971). One or more serum samples from each patient were assayed for HBsAg.

Liver specimens

Liver biopsies from seven patients were taken on the basis of overt liver abnormalities. No attempt was made to obtain liver tissues from the remaining patients who were without clinical manifestations of liver disease.

Results

Table 9.1 shows the frequency of HBsAg in the serum as well as in the kidney of patients with glomerulonephritis. Of 66 kidney specimens, 34 were histologically diagnosed as various forms of glomerulonephritis. A higher rate of positivity was obtained in tissue (42%) than in the serum (30%). As a whole 22% of the kidney biopsies were HBsAg positive. The highest number of cases had membranoproliferative glomerulonephritis (14 of 34). HBsAg was demonstrated in 5 of 7 cases of membranous, 6 of 14 cases of membranoproliferative, 2 of 8 cases of intracapillary proliferative glomerulonephritis and 1 of 3 cases of minimal change.

Table 9.1 Incidence of HBsAg in patients with various types of glomerulonephritis

Histological diagnosis	No.	HBsAg in serum	HBsAg in biopsy
1. GLOMERULONEPHRITIS			
Membranoproliferative	14	4	6
Membranous	7	4	5
Intracapillary proliferative	8	1	2
Focal local glomerulonephritis	2	—	—
Minimal changes	3	1	1
Total	34	10 (30%)	14 (42%)
2. MISCELLANEOUS	32	—	—
TOTAL	66	10	14 (22%)

Immune complex deposition in relationship to HBsAg demonstration

Table 9.2 summarizes the patterns of immune complex deposition in HBsAg positive as well as in HBsAg negative glomerulonephritis. Of 34 cases, 32 showed variable amounts of immunoglobulins and complement in the glomeruli. Immune complexes could be demonstrated in all 14 cases

Table 9.2 Patterns of immune complex deposition in HBsAg positive and HBsAg negative glomerulonephritis

	No.	G*	A*	M*	GA	GM	AM	GAM	B₁C
HBsAg positive glomerulonephritis									
Membranoproliferative	6	1	—	—	2	1	—	2	6
Membranous	5	3	—	—	—	—	2	—	5
Intracapillary proliferative	2	—	—	—	1	1	—	—	2
Minimal changes**	1	—	—	—	1	—	—	—	1
Total	14	4	—	—	4	2	2	2	14
HBsAg negative glomerulonephritis									
Membranoproliferative	8	—	2	1	—	—	4	—	8
Membranous	2	—	—	—	—	—	1	1	2
Intracapillary proliferative	6	—	1	1	—	—	3	—	5
Focal local	2	—	—	—	—	—	—	1	1
Minimal changes**	2	—	—	—	—	—	—	1	2
Total	20	—	3	2	—	—	8	3	18

* G IgG: A IgA; M IgM
** only a faint reaction was obtained for immunoglobulins and complement components

with HBsAg. HBsAg was found to be deposited in the same sites as immunoglobulin and complement. A dissociated pattern among the components of immune complexes was rarely observed. The glomerular depositions were granular and lumpy, distributed diffusely in the capillary walls (Figure 9.1). However, segmental positivity was also observed. HBsAg immune complexes were also localized in the mesangium. The characteristic glomerular deposition patterns of immune complexes were in conformity with the histological diagnosis. In the HBsAg positive group IgG alone or in combination was more frequently observed than IgA or IgM, whereas IgA and/or IgM were predominant components of immune complexes in the HBsAg negative group (Table 9.2).

Spectrum of liver diseases in HBsAg positive glomerulonephritis

From the 14 HBsAg positive cases, liver biopsies were available for examination from 7; of these 7 patients, 4 specimens were taken prior to the clinical diagnosis of glomerulonephritis. From these 7 patients, 5 had cirrhosis (3 less active; 2 active) and 2 had CAH (Table 9.3). Liver disease was present in each group of glomerulonephritis (3 in membrano-proliferative; 2 in membranous; 1 in intracapillary proliferative; 1 in minimal changes). Frozen sections from 4 liver specimens (3 cirrhosis;

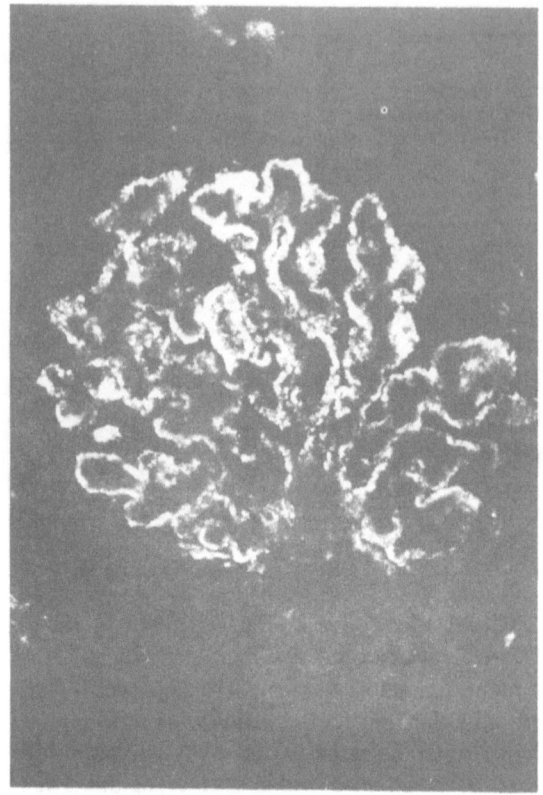

Figure 9.1 Kidney biopsy from a patient with membranous glomerulonephritis. HBsAg is demonstrated in the capillary walls. The fluorescence is strong and coarsely granular in character. Similar characteristic deposition of complement and IgG were observed in the same sites (× 230)

1 CAH) were available for the detection of HBV components, VCF and immunoglobulin deposition (Table 9.3). Cytoplasmic and membrane-localized HBsAg could be demonstrated in 3 cases of active liver disease (2 cirrhosis; 1 CAH). HBcAg, VCF and IgG were observed mostly in the hepatocytic nuclei and rarely in the cytoplasmic periphery or cell membrane. HBcAg, VCF and IgG were not demonstrated in the single case of less active cirrhosis which showed diffuse distribution of HBsAg only in the cytoplasm.

Table 9.3 Spectrum of liver histology observed in 7 cases of HBsAg positive glomerulonephritis

Types of glomerulonephritis	No.	Cirrhosis		CAH
		Less active	Active	
Membranoproliferative	3	1*	1*	1
Membranous	2	1	—	1*
Intracapillary proliferative	1	1	—	—
Minimal changes	1	—	1*	—
Total	7	3	2	2

*Frozen sections examined for HBV components, VCF and immunoglobulins

Discussion

The present study further confirms the previously reported association between HBV and glomerulonephritis (Combes et al., 1971; Myers et al., 1973; Krieser et al., 1974; Kohler et al., 1974; Brzosko et al., 1974). In this series the frequency of HBsAg positivity is 42%; this is slightly lower than that observed (56%) in Warsaw (Brzosko et al., 1974) and slightly higher than that (23%) reported from South Africa (Vos et al., 1973). However, it should be emphasized that some kidney biopsies were obtained from haemodialysis patients who have a higher attack rate than non-dialysed renal patients; so the incidence of 42% may not represent the true incidence of HBsAg in this group of glomerulonephritis patients. HBsAg was demonstrated in the kidney of all 10 seropositive cases and in 4 additional patients who were seronegative for HBsAg. These findings are similar to those reported by other investigators (Knieser et al., 1974; Brzosko et al., 1974; Conte and Fournie, 1975). The data reported in the literature are compared in Table 9.4.

Table 9.4 Comparison of results on the HBsAg positivity in kidney and serum of patients with glomerulonephritis

Authors	HBsAg positivity (%) in	
	Kidney	Serum
Brzosko et al. (1974)	56	50
Conte and Fournie (1975)	31	0
Nagy et al. (1978)	16	16
Present study	42	30

The characteristic granular and lumpy deposition of HBsAg in the capillary walls and/or mesangium along with the presence of immunoglobulins and complement strongly suggests the formation of HBsAg immune complexes in the glomerulus. This has been observed only in 42% of the cases – the remaining 58% also had demonstrable immunoglobulins and complement but no HBsAg was observed. These findings support the hypothesis of Dixon (1968) and Oldstone and Dixon (1971) that most cases of glomerulonephritis are of immunological origin. The present and the previous investigations show that multiple histological types of glomerulonephritis are observed in association with HBV infection. Based on these findings, a parallel can be drawn with the reported experimental investigations where different glomerular lesions developed after the injection of bovine serum albumin as antigen. This stimulated antibody production with formation of immune complexes (Dixon et al., 1961) (Germuth and Rodriguez, 1973) in various concentration and size.

Although HBsAg was demonstrated in the glomeruli, the exact role of HBV in the development of glomerulonephritis remains obscure. Anti-HBs (supposed to be one of the components of the immune complexes) was rarely detected in the serum of patients with HBsAg positive glomerulonephritis as well as hepatitis (Chapter 5). Nevertheless, several studies dealing with the various extrahepatic manifestations of hepatitis B (Chapter 10) (Gyorkey et al., 1975), reported low titres of anti-HBs in the cryoprecipitate made from the serum but rarely in the whole blood. In the present study circulating anti-HBs is still under investigation.

The link between chronic liver disease and glomerulonephritis was recognized long ago (Baxter and Ashworth, 1946; Patek et al., 1951). A variety of renal lesions was described (Callard et al., 1975) in patients with biopsy proven alcoholic liver diseases without circulating HBsAg. Therefore it can be questioned whether immune complex deposits in the glomerulus are the primary aetiological factor in the development of glomerulonephritis or whether they are simply an epiphenomenon. However, Gyorkey et al. (1975) could induce immune complex nephritis in baboons by inoculating human plasma rich in Dane particles. Glomerular lesions in these animals were comparable to those observed in the early stage of acute hepatitis B (Eknoyan et al., 1972). Intranuclear virus particles (26 nm), were observed in the hepatocytes. These findings may support the idea that HBV may be one of the aetiological agents of glomerulonephretis.

The spectrum of liver histology in HBsAg positive glomerulonephritis was not studied systematically. In previous investigations, liver histology showed the picture of chronic active forms of liver disease (Combes et al., 1971; Knieser et al., 1974). However, Brzosko et al. (1974) did not observe overt liver abnormalities in children with HBsAg positive glomerulonephritis. In the present investigation, liver biopsy was taken only in cases with clinical signs of liver disease. Of the seven, 5 showed fully developed cirrhosis and 2 had CAH. The intrahepatic expression patterns of HBV components were in conformity with the histological diagnosis. Immune complexes specific for HBcAg but not for HBsAg were observed in the hepatocytes. Therefore it is evident that extrahepatic tissue injury is probably caused by the deposition of HBsAg immune complexes but the exact role of these complexes in the development of the associated liver pathology remains to be elucidated.

References

Baxter, J. H. and Ashworth, C. T. (1946). Renal lesions in portal cirrhosis. *Arch. Path.*, **41**, 476

Brzosko, W. J., Krawczynski, K., Nazarewicz, T., Morzycka, M. and Nowoslawski, A. (1974). Glomerulonephritis associated with hepatitis B surface antigen immune complexes in children. *Lancet*, **2**, 477

Callard, P., Feldmann, G., Prandi, D., Belair, M. F., Mandet, C., Weiss, Y., Druet, P., Benhamou, J. P. and Bariety, J. (1975). Immune complex type glomerulonephritis in cirrhosis of the liver. *Am. J. Path.*, **80**, 329

Combes, B., Stastny, P., Shorey, J., Eigenbrodt, E. H., Barrera, A., Hull, A. R. and Carter, N. W. (1971). Glomerulonephritis with deposition of Australia antigen–antibody complexes in glomerular basement membrane. *Lancet*, **2**, 234

Conte, J. J. and Fournie, G. J. (1975). Antigène Australia et glomérulonéphrites. *La Nouvelle Presse Médicale*, **4**, 429

Dixon, F. J. (1968). The pathogenesis of glomerulonephritis (Editorial). *Am. Med. J.*, **44**, 493

Dixon, F. J., Feldman, J. D. and Vazquez, J. J. (1961). Experimental glomerulonephritis: the pathogensis of a laboratory model resembling the spectrum of human glomerulo nephritis. *J. Exp. Med.*, **113**, 899

Eknoyan, G., Gyorkey, F., Dichoso, C., Martinez-Maldonado, M., Suki, W. N. and Gyorkey, P. (1972). Renal morphological and immunological changes associated with viral hepatitis. *Kidney International*, **1**, 413

Germuth, F. G. and Rodriguez, E. (1973). Immune complex deposite glomerular disease. In *Immunopathology of the Renal Glomerulus*, pp. 1–56. (Boston: Little Brown and Co.)

Gyorkey, F., Hollinger, F. B., Eknoyan, G., Mirkovic, R., Dreesman, G. R., Gyorkey, P., Voss, W. R. and Melnick, J. L. (1975). Immune complex glomerulonephritis, intra nuclear particles in hepatocytes and *in vivo* clearance rates in sub-human primates inoculated with HBsAg containing plasma. *Exp. Mol. Path.*, **22**, 350

Habib, R. and Kleinknecht, C. (1971). The primary nephrotic syndrome of childhood: classification and clinicopathologic study of 406 cases. *Path. A;* **6**, 417

Knieser, M. R., Jenis, E. H., Lowenthal, D. T., Bancroft, W. H., Burns, W. and Shalhoub, R. (1974). Pathogenesis of renal disease associated with viral hepatitis. *Arch. Path.*, **97**, 193

Kohler, P. F., Cronin, R. E., Hammond, W. S., Olin, D. and Carr, R. I. (1974). Chronic membranous glomerulonephritis caused by hepatitis B antigen antibody immune complexes. *Ann. Int. Med.*, **81**, 448

Myers, B. D., Griffel, B., Naveh, D., Jankielowitz, T. and Klajman, A. (1973). Membrano-proliferative glomerulonephritis associated with persistent viral hepatitis. *Am. J. Clin. Path.*, **59**, 222

Nagy, J., Bajtai, G., Brasch, H., Sule, T., Ambrus, M., Deak, G. and Hamori, A. (1978). HBsAg in renal disease. *Lancet*, **2**, 315

Oldstone, M. B. A. and Dixon, F. J. (1971). Immune complex disease in viral infections. *J. Exp. Med.*, **134**, 32

Patek, A. J., Seegal, D. and Bevans, M. (1951). The co-existence of cirrhosis of the liver and glomerulonephritis: report of 14 cases. *Am. J. Med. Sci.*, **221**, 77

Vos, G. H., Grobbelaar, B. G. and Milner, L. V. (1973). A possible relationship between persistent hepatitis B antigenaemia and renal disease in Southern African Bantu. *S. Afr. Med. J.*, **47**, 911

PART IV
Speculations and hypothesis concerning the pathogenesis of hepatitis B

10
Possible mechanisms of tissue injury in hepatitis B virus infection

In the previous chapters HBV antigens have been shown to be associated with both intrahepatic and extrahepatic diseases. The morphological appearances and immunopathological abnormalities suggest that immunological processes may be involved and that host immune responses to the viral antigens may determine tissue damage.

At least five major types of hypersensitivity reactions are involved in tissue injury (Table 10.1). In the light of the present findings and the data from the literature this chapter discusses the participation of the most probable immunological reactions in the causation of tissue damage in HBV infection.

Table 10.1 Types of hypersensitivity reactions

Immunological reactions		Mediators
Type I	Anaphylactic or immediate hypersensitivity	Mast cells, vasoactive amines
Type II	Cytotoxic or cytolytic	Macrophages, complement
Type III	Immune complex	Complement, B cells, hydrolytic enzymes from polymorphs
Type IV	Cell mediated immunity	Lymphokines, T cells
Type V	Antibody dependent cellular cytotoxicity	K cells

TYPE I REACTIONS (ANAPHYLACTIC OR IMMEDIATE HYPERSENSITIVITY)

Type I reactions are produced by pharmacologically active substances released from basophils and mast cells following reactions between antigen and specific antibody absorbed to the mast cell membrane. The role of this type of reaction has not been adequately investigated in hepatitis B. Recent studies reported an increase in serum IgE values (Van Epps *et al.*, 1975; Joske *et al.*, 1976) and the liver mast cells in patients with chronic aggressive hepatitis (Kurokawa, 1976). However, in these studies the results were not correlated with the HBV antigen status of the patients. Moreover no correlation seemed to exist between the level of circulating IgE and signs of hepatocellular damage. The increased tissue mast cells seen as part of the mononuclear cell infiltration in the portal tract and the increased IgE levels in the serum as a consequence of the generally increased immunoglobulin production.

TYPE II REACTIONS (CYTOTOXIC OR CYTOLYTIC)

Type II reactions are mediated by the combination of antibodies (mainly auto-antibodies of IgG or IgM classes) with antigens present in the target cell membrane or with circulating antigens or haptens absorbed to the target cell surfaces. Cytolysis occurs either by phagocytosis or by activation of the whole complement cascade.

Tissue antibodies

A variety of tissue antibodies have been found in patients with acute and chronic hepatitis. They include ANF, AMA, SMA, bile canalicular antibodies and antiglomerular basement antibodies. These antibodies however are not liver specific and do not seem to correlate with the severity of the disease (Doniach, 1970); their cytotoxicity on liver cells in culture is controversial (Paronetto *et al.*, 1973). Moreover complement has not been observed at the site of tissue damage (Paronetto, 1973). These antibodies may not have any pathogenetic role in hepatitis B as they are more frequently found in HBsAg negative than in HBsAg positive cases (Bulkley *et al.*, 1970; Wright, 1970; Dawkins and Joske, 1973).

Liver specific proteins

Two liver specific antigens, a cytoplasmic protein and a macromolecular, membrane-localized, low density lipoprotein (LSP) have been identified by Meyer zum Buschenfelde and Miescher (1972). LSP has been found to be organ specific but not species specific (Hopf *et al.*, 1974). As the antigen is a normal constituent of the cell membrane and is shown to induce chronic liver disease in rabbits (Meyer zum Buschenfelde *et al.*, 1972) (after injection of the antigen in Freund's adjuvants) a concept of autoimmune liver disease, the existence of which has long been suspected, emerged rather quickly. This concept promoted the search for the specific antibody (liver cell membrane autoantibody LMA) in the serum of patients with various hepatic and non-hepatic disorders (Hopf *et al.*, 1976; Tage-Jensen *et al.*, 1977).

By indirect fluorescence Hopf *et al.* (1976) detected LMA in the sera of 7 of 10 HBsAg negative CAH patients. Membrane-localized IgG could be demonstrated in isolated hepatocytes obtained from all 10 patients. Membrane bound IgG was also localized in 15 of 19 HBsAg seropositive cases without circulating LMA. However, in HBsAg negative cases IgG was deposited linearly in the cell membrane in contrast to the granular deposition observed in HBsAg positive cases. Based on the absence of circulating anti-HBs in HBsAg positive patients, it was suggested that the deposited IgG may be an antibody against an unknown antigen (neo-antigen) produced in the hepatocytic membrane after HBV infection. However, neither serum anti-HBc nor hepatic HBcAg was investigated in those patients. In a similar but more extended study Tage-Jensen *et al.* (1977) have reported a higher prevalence (approx. 50%) of LMA in HBsAg negative CAH (including non-alcoholic cirrhosis) than in HBsAg positive CAH (5%). Therefore it seems that LSP or the putative antigen of LMA may play a significant role in the pathogenesis of HBsAg negative chronic hepatitis. However, it is not entirely clear at the present time whether 'LMA' and 'anti-LSP' are strictly identical.

TYPE III REACTIONS (IMMUNE COMPLEX TYPE)

Type III reactions are initiated by the formation of antigen–antibody complexes and fixation of complement at the site of antigen–antibody deposition. Tissue damage is mainly caused by the liberation of hydrolytic enzymes from attracted polymorphonuclear leukocytes.

HBV antigens immune complexes in the pathogenesis of hepatitis B

Infection with HBV is usually associated with the production of specific antibodies to both HBsAg (i.e. anti-HBs) and HBcAg (i.e. anti-HBc).

The prevalence of serum anti-HBs in the presence of HBsAg has consistently been found to be low in both acute and chronic hepatitis B. It was detected in 80% of the individuals following disappearance of circulating HBsAg and during subsidence of liver disease (Barker *et al.*, 1973). Serial

135

serum examination in subjects with experimentally induced hepatitis B (Bulkley *et al.*, 1970; Hoofnagle *et al.*, 1975) could detect anti-HBs only long after the disappearance of circulating HBsAg. Moreover, the presence of circulating HBsAg immune complexes in patients with polyarteritis nodosa could not be correlated with the severity of the hepatocellular damage (Prince and Trepo, 1971; Trepo *et al.*, 1974). Nevertheless such immune complexes have been detected in fulminant hepatitis B (Trepo *et al.*, 1976; Woolf *et al.*, 1976), and it has been suggested that these immune complexes may be cytopathic. However, infusion of serum containing anti-HBs did not promote liver cell necrosis in HBsAg positive patients with chronic hepatitis (Reed *et al.*, 1973; Kohler *et al.*, 1974).

At the cellular level, only membrane-localized HBsAg could be correlated with both histological (piecemeal necrosis) and clinical (high serum transaminases) signs of active disease (Ray *et al.*, 1976). Immunoglobulin was rarely observed in the cell membrane and never in the cytoplasm. Although membrane-localized IgG was demonstrated in isolated hepatocytes obtained from HBsAg positive CAH patients, no anti-HBs could be detected in their blood (Hopf *et al.*, 1976). Therefore the role of HBsAg immune complexes in the pathogenesis of hepatitis B remains to be clarified.

Specific antibody responses to the HBcAg have been observed consistently following HBV infection (Hoofnagle *et al.*, 1973; 1974; Barker *et al.*, 1975). Anti-HBc was detected in 100% of the sera of HBsAg positive patients but only in a few HBsAg negative patients (Chapter 5). It was present in 82% of blood donors implicated in transmission of hepatitis B (Hoofnagle *et al.*, 1974). Hoofnagle *et al.* (1973) reported high titres of circulating anti-HBc in 'chronic HBsAg carriers'. Chronic carriers were defined as persons who had detectable HBsAg for a minimum period of six months. Neither the liver histology nor the intrahepatic expression patterns of HBV antigens were investigated in those 'carriers'. Recently however, higher titres of anti-HBc have been observed more frequently in patients with chronic aggressive hepatitis B compared to the less aggressive forms (Hadziyannis and Karvountvis, 1976; Endo *et al.*, 1978). High titres have also been observed in fully developed acute hepatitis B as well as in the exacerbation stage of chronic hepatitis B (our own observation, unpublished) indicating a certain parallelism between high titres of circulating anti-HBc and signs of disease activity.

The possible role of HBcAg immune complexes has received limited attention, maybe due to the frequent presence of anti-HBc in HBsAg carriers, in HBsAg positive and in HBsAg negative hepatitis. In experimental hepatitis B (Krugman *et al.*, 1974; Hoofnagle *et al.*, 1975), it has consistently been observed that anti-HBc appeared in the serum usually after the appearance of HBsAg and just prior to or at the onset of clinical hepatitis. This has been correlated with the formation of *in vitro* HBcAg immune complex in the liver (Chapter 7). The high prevalence of such an immune complex could also be correlated with the signs of hepatocellular necrosis in chronic aggressive forms of hepatitis B (Chapter 5).

Although complement binding could be readily demonstrated after adding it *in vitro*, for some unknown reasons it has not yet been demonstrated in hepatic tissue as such. Serum complement levels decrease in various liver diseases but this could not be evaluated properly because the liver produces certain components of the complement system. Therefore lower values may indicate decreased hepatic synthesis as well as complement consumption by immune complexes. However serum C1q (which is of extrahepatic origin) has been found to be unaltered in chronic liver diseases (Finlayson *et al.*, 1972). The mechanism of the cytolytic activity of this supposed HBcAg immune complex is not yet known but the paradox is that polymorphonuclear leukocytes, the hallmark of immune complex induced tissue damage, are rarely observed in the liver specimens obtained from hepatitis patients. Nevertheless one could speculate that HBcAg immune complexes may be cytopathic independent of neutrophil accumulation as has been observed in some immune complex induced renal diseases (Henson, 1971).

Extrahepatic manifestations of HBV infection

An increasing amount of evidence suggests that HBV infection is associated with the production of tissue damage outside the liver. The most common sites involved are skin, joints, arteries, arterioles and renal glomeruli. Table 10.2 summarizes the various extrahepatic diseases reported in association with HBV infection. Immunological mechanisms, especially immune complex deposition, appear to be responsible for these extrahepatic manifestations. Each pathological entity is discussed in the following paragraphs.

Table 10.2 Extrahepatic manifestations of HBV infection

Diseases	Authors
Polyarteritis nodosa	Gocke *et al.* (1970); Trepo *et al.* (1970)
Arthritis	Alpert *et al.* (1971); Onion *et al.* (1971)
Glomerulonephritis	Combes *et al.* (1971)
Infantile papular acrodermatitis	Gianotti (1973)
Polymyalgia rheumatica	Bacon *et al.* (1975)
Guillain Barré syndrome	Ng *et al.* (1975)
Peripheral neuropathy	Farivar *et al.* (1976)
Essential mixed cryoglobulinaemia	Levo *et al.* (1977)

Serum sickness-like syndrome in acute hepatitis B

Urticaria, skin eruptions, polyarthralgia and even frank arthiritis have long been recognized as various prodromal symptoms of acute hepatitis (Marner, 1952). The incidental discovery of the association between HBsAg and arthritis (Alpert *et al.*, 1971; Onion *et al.*, 1971) has drawn renewed attention to this problem. The syndrome appears in the incubation period or in the early stage of both HBsAg positive and HBsAg negative hepatitis (Fernandez and McCarthy, 1971), and usually disappears at the onset of clinical symptoms. Serum complement level is depressed in the early stage of the disease when HBsAg titres are high, suggesting formation of immune complexes in antigen excess. Recently several studies (Wands *et al.*, 1975; McIntosh *et al.*, 1976) have shown that although anti-HBs is rarely detected in the serum of patients with HBsAg associated arthritis, cryo-precipitates isolated from serum of such patients contain HBsAg, anti-HBs and complement. Similar cryoprecipitates but without complement have been found in patients with acute hepatitis B without arthritis. Wands *et al.* (1975) have further shown the presence of complement fixing IgG_1 and IgG_3 in the cryoprecipitates and C3 activator fragment of the properdin complex in the serum of arthritis patients with circulating HBsAg. These findings suggest the participation of both classical and alternate pathways of complement activation in the pathogenesis of arthritis in hepatitis B.

Polyarteritis nodosa associated with HBV infection

Gocke *et al.* (1970) and Trepo and Thivolet (1970) first described poly-arteritis nodosa in association with HBV infection. This has since been confirmed by several other authors (Gerber *et al.*, 1972; Baker *et al.*, 1972; Heathcote *et al.*, 1972). The frequency of HBsAg antigenaemia may be as high as 30 to 40% in vasculitis (Gocke *et al.*, 1970). Patients often present with fever and may subsequently develop hypertension, renal dysfunctions and peripheral neuropathies. HBsAg persists for long periods of time and a depression of the blood C3 level is noted in the acute stage of the disease. Small and medium sized blood vessels show fibrinoid necrosis and peri-vascular mononuclear cell infiltration. Muscle and kidney biopsies show deposition of HBsAg, immunoglobulins (IgM or IgG) and C3 in granular patterns, compatible with the presence of cytopathic immune complexes.

The spectrum of liver disease in HBsAg associated vasculitis has not yet been studied systematically. In an elaborate retrospective investigation Sergent *et al.* (1976) investigated the natural evolution of vasculitis in patients with HBsAg antigenaemia. Of the 9 patients, 6 showed initially either acute or chronic hepatitis followed by vasculitis. Two of the remaining

3 first had signs of vasculitis followed by chronic hepatitis. Therefore it seems that polyarteritis nodosa may be a secondary phenomenon in HBV infection. However, Trepo *et al* (1974) in a survey of 55 patients with biopsy documented polyarteritis nodosa, reported 69% positivity either for HBsAg and/or anti-HBs. HBsAg immune complexes in serum were demonstrated in 66% of patients but their presence could not be correlated with severity of liver disease.

Glomerulonephritis associated with HBV infection

The incidence of HBV infection in glomerulonephritis and its immuno-pathology have been described in Chapter 9.

Other extrahepatic diseases associated with HBV infection

Recently polymyalgia rheumatica (Bacon *et al.*, 1975), Guillain Barré syndrome (Ng *et al.*, 1975), peripheral neuropathies (Farivar *et al.*, 1976) and essential mixed cryoglobulinaemia (Levo *et al.*, 1977) have been described in association with HBV infection. HBsAg immune complexes have been demonstrated in the serum of such patients. In polymyalgia rheumatica, although no circulating HBsAg was detected, anti-HBs was found in the blood with high frequency.

Infantile papular acrodermatitis (Gianotti, 1973) has also been found to be associated with HBV infection (subtype ayw). Patients show minimal liver dysfunctions. The immunopathological mechanisms involved in this disease remain to be elucidated.

TYPE IV REACTIONS (CELL MEDIATED IMMUNITY – CMI)

Type IV reactions occur as a result of the interaction between sensitized lymphocytes and specific antigens, usually present in the cell surface. These reactions are antibody and complement independent. Tissue damage is mediated by the release of lymphokines, by direct cytotoxicity or both.

The characteristic predominant lymphocytic infiltration (Review, 1977) in the liver of hepatitis patients is a sufficient reason to consider the possible role of CMI in the pathogenesis of hepatitis B. To date, the accumulated data, using various parameters to assess the CMI, are confusing and sometimes even contradictory. However, to put the informations in a meaningful order, the basic data obtained in hepatitis will be discussed.

Skin tests

Intradermal injections of antigens and sensitization with dichlorobenzene has been used to assess CMI in hepatitis patients. No alteration of reactivity was observed in HBsAg positive or HBsAg negative acute hepatitis compared to controls (Sodomann *et al.*, 1974); however, impaired skin sensitization has been reported in chronic hepatitis (Toh *et al.*, 1973; Sodomann *et al.*, 1974) indicating depressed cellular immunity.

Peripheral and hepatic T and B cells

There is almost general agreement on the decrease of the absolute number of circulating T lymphocytes in both HBsAg positive and HBsAg negative acute and chronic hepatitis (De Horatius *et al.*, 1974; Thomas *et al.*, 1976; Degast *et al.*, 1976; Ishimaru *et al.*, 1976; Aldershvile *et al.*, 1977). However, Wicks *et al.* (1975) and Galili *et al.* (1975) have shown normal values in such patients; on the other hand, Miller *et al.* (1977) have reported a decrease of such cells in HBsAg positive chronic hepatitis and a normal number in the HBsAg negative group. In healthy HBsAg carriers and in the resolving stage of acute hepatitis (De Horatius *et al.*, 1974; Thomas *et al.*, 1976; Ishimaru *et al.*, 1976) the population of circulating T lymphocytes is not different from controls.

Null cells (cells without surface immunoglobulins and not identified by T cell markers) are increased in both HBsAg positive and HBsAg negative acute and chronic hepatitis (Thomas *et al.*, 1976; Aldershvile *et al.*, 1977). Their population is found to be normal in CPH and HBsAg carriers (Thomas *et al.*, 1976).

In liver specimens, the number of T cells is reported to be higher in both HBsAg positive and HBsAg negative chronic hepatitis (as has also been seen in alcoholic liver disease and in primary biliary cirrhosis) than in inactive cirrhosis and CPH (Husby *et al.*, 1975; Aldershvile *et al.*, 1977; Sanchez-Tapias *et al.*, 1977). These findings are in contradiction to those of Miller *et al.* (1977) who have observed a significantly higher number of T cells in HBsAg associated chronic hepatitis than in the HBsAg negative group.

Information available to date shows an inverse relationship between the circulating and hepatic T lymphocytes in patients with both HBsAg associated and HBsAg negative hepatitis. The exact cause of the peripheral lymphocytopenia and tissular lymphocytosis is not known. It may be related either to the presence of single or multiple serum inhibitors (Husby *et al.*, 1975; Chisari and Edgington, 1975) which may influence T cell rosette formation or may be the result of sequestration of peripheral T cells into the liver (Miller et al., 1977).

There is no significant alteration in the circulating B cell population among patients with HBsAg positive or HBsAg negative hepatitis or with HBsAg carriers compared to the normal controls (Thomas et al., 1976; Ishimaru et al., 1976; Aldershvile et al., 1977; Miller et al., 1977; Sanchez-Tapias et al., 1977). The above findings contradict De Horatius et al. (1974) who have observed a significant increase of peripheral B lymphocytes in both HBsAg positive and HBsAg negative acute and chronic hepatitis. In the liver specimens B cells are found to be equally increased in both type B and non-B acute and chronic hepatitis (Aldershvile et al., 1977; Sanchez-Tapias et al., 1977). However Miller et al. (1977) have reported a higher number of such cells in HBsAg negative hepatitis than in the HBsAg positive group.

In vitro lymphocyte stimulation by HBV antigens and mitogens

Blast transformation of sensitized lymphocytes by antigens or mitogens has been commonly used to assess cellular immunity. Lymphocyte stimulation by semipurified HBsAg has been observed in patients recovering from acute hepatitis B (Pettigrew et al., 1972; Degast et al., 1973; Laiwah et al., 1973; Warnatz, 1974; Sodomann et al., 1974). These results may suggest that CMI is necessary to clear the virus. In fully developed acute hepatitis, lymphocyte stimulation is found to be variable (Sodomann et al., 1974; Warnatz, 1974. It has not been demonstrated in HBsAg carriers (Pettigrew et al., 1972; Sodomann et al., 1974). Nevertheless, Warnatz (1974) has observed an increased response in a few cases with both HBsAg positive and HBsAg negative hepatitis.

In vitro stimulation of lymphocytes by HBcAg in hepatitis patients remains to be investigated.

A depression of phytohemagglutinin (PHA) induced lymphocyte transformation has been noted in HBsAg positive as well as in HBsAg negative acute hepatitis (Newble et al., 1975; Thestrup-Pedersen et al., 1976; Sato et al., 1976). As in normal HBsAg carriers, no alteration was observed in the resolving stage of acute hepatitis B (Degast et al., 1973; Warnatz, 1974; Sato et al., 1976). In chronic hepatitis with or without circulating HBsAg, the results obtained are very variable; PHA has been found to stimulate (Tolentino et al., 1974) to depress (Pettigrew et al., 1972) or to produce no change of reaction (Sodomann et al., 1974; Warnatz, 1974; Sato et al., 1976; Thestrup-Pedersen et al., 1976).

In vitro inhibition of leukocyte migration by HBV antigens

Inhibition of leukocyte migration by antigen has been considered to be one of the specific tests to determine cellular immunity. Patients with acute hepatitis B show inhibition of leukocyte migration in the presence of purified or semipurified HBsAg (Dudley et al., 1972; Irwin et al., 1974; Gerber et al., 1974; Demura et al., 1975). In the resolving stage of acute hepatitis, the reaction becomes normal. However, these latter findings are in contradiction to the observation of Laiwah et al. (1973) and Frei et al. (1973) who have reported inhibition of migration in such patients. In patients with both HBsAg positive and HBsAg negative chronic hepatitis, purified HBsAg failed to inhibit leukocyte migration (Demura et al., 1975). These data are again at variance with the findings of Irwin et al. (1974) and Dudley et al (1972) who have shown migration inhibition in some patients with chronic hepatitis B. Leukocyte migration has not yet been studied with HBcAg.

Lymphocyte cytotoxicity in vitro

In vitro target cell death after addition of sensitized lymphocytes is considered as a correlate of T cell immunity. It has recently been used to determine the mechanism of liver cell injury in both acute and chronic hepatitis (Thomson et al., 1974; Wands and Isselbacher, 1975; Paronetto (Thomson et al., 1974), homologous (Wands and Isselbacher, 1975) or autologous liver cells (Paronetto and Vernace, 1975) than to control lymphocytes. However, this phenomenon is not disease specific. It may represent merely a mechanism of cell killing, as cytotoxic activity has been observed in HBsAg positive and HBsAg negative acute and chronic hepatitis (Thomson et al., 1974; (Wands and Isselbacher, 1975; Paronetto and Vernace, 1975) and in primary biliary cirrhosis (Paronetto and Vernace, 1975; Geubel et al., 1976).

Lymphocyte cytotoxicity may represent a normal defence mechanism of the host and its impairment may be responsible for the persistence of the disease (Dudley et al., 1972). Cytotoxicity is inhibited by immunosuppressive agents and by inhibiting factors present in autologous or homologous sera (Wands and Isselbacher, 1975; Paronetto and Vernace, 1975). However, spontaneous cytotoxicity has been observed in patients with CAH and primary biliary cirrhosis (Geubel et al., 1976).

TYPE V REACTION
(ANTIBODY DEPENDENT CELLULAR CYTOTOXICITY)

Type V reaction is mediated by unsensitized lymphocytes designated 'K' cells, which do not have T or B cell characteristics; they bind with the activated Fc portion of the specific antibody complexed with the antigen present in the target cell membrane and cause cytolysis independent of complement.

Information on the participation of this reaction in the pathogenesis of hepatitis B is scanty. Recently K cell cytotoxicity has been suggested in the development of both HBsAg positive and HBsAg negative chronic hepatitis (Cochrane et al., 1976; Kawanishi, 1977). The precise character and role of the K cells is still unclear and more investigation has to be performed to come to definite conclusions (Mikulski, 1976).

GENETIC FACTORS IN HEPATITIS

Recognition of the link between selected histocompatibility antigens (HLA system) and some specific pathological entities has drawn attention to the genetic constitution as an important determinant of some acquired diseases. Blumberg et al. (1969; 1970) first proposed that the distribution and persistence of the chronic antigen carrier state were determined by genetic factors of the host. This hypothesis has recently been tested on individuals with hepatitis B. There is increasing evidence for the high prevalence of HLA-B8 phenotypes in HBsAg negative chronic hepatitis (Mackey and Morris, 1972; Galbraith et al., 1974; Freudenberg et al., 1977). Such phenotypes have been found to be in normal proportions in the HBsAg positive group (Galbraith et al., 1974). HLA-B8 has also been associated with HBsAg positive renal dialysis patients who ultimately cleared the antigen (Jungers et al., 1975; Descamps et al., 1977). Recently Hillis et al. (1977) have reported a high prevalence of BW15 in transient and BW17 in persistent HBsAg antigenaemia in renal dialysis or transplant patients. These data seem to be promising; however, further investigation is necessary in order to firmly establish the association between genetic factors and chronic hepatitis.

References

Aldershvile. J., Dietrichson. O., Hardt. F. and Nielsen. O. J. (1977). Circulating T and B lymphocytes and immunoglobulin containing cells in the liver in chronic active liver disease. *Acta Path. Microbiol. Scand. Sect. C*, **85**. 26

Alpert. E., Isselbacher. K. J. and Schur. P. H. (1971). The pathogenesis of arthritis associated with viral hepatitis. *N. Engl. J. Med.*, **285**. 185

Bacon. P. A., Doherty. S. M. and Zuckerman. A. J. (1975). Hepatitis B antibody in polymyalgia rheumatica. *Lancet*, **2**. 476

Baker. A. L., Kaplan. M. M., Benz. W. C., Sidel. J. S. and Wolfe. H. J. (1972). Poly-arteritis associated with Australia antigen positive hepatitis. *Gastroenterology*, **62**. 105

HEPATITIS B VIRUS ANTIGENS IN TISSUES

Barker, L. F., Peterson, M. R., Shulman, N. R. and Murray, R. (1973). Antibody responses in viral hepatitis type B. *JAMA*, **223**, 1005

Barker, L. F., Maynard, J. E., Purcell, R. H., Hoofnagle, J. H., Berquist, K. R. and London, W. T. (1975). Viral hepatitis type B in experimental animals. *Am. J. Med. Sci.*, **270**, 189

Blumberg, B. S., Friedlaender, J. S., Woodside, A., Sutnick, A. I. and London, W. T. (1969). Hepatitis and Australia antigen: autosomal recessive inheritance of susceptibility to infection in humans. *Proc. Natl. Acad. Sci. USA*, **62**, 1108

Blumberg, B. S., Sutnick, A. I. and London, W. T. (1970). Australia antigen as a hepatitis virus: variation in host response. *Am. J. Med.*, **48**, 1

Bulkley, B. H., Heizer, W. D., Goldfinger, S. E., Isselbacher, K. J. and Shulman, N. R. (1970). Distinctions in chronic active hepatitis based on circulating hepatitis-associated antigen. *Lancet*, **2**, 1323

Chisari, F. V. and Edgington, T. S. (1975). Lymphocyte E rosette inhibitory factor: a regulatory serum lipoprotein. *J. Exp. Med.*, **142**, 1092

Cochrane, A. M. G., Moussouros, A., Thomson, A. D., Eddleston, A. L. W. F. and Williams, R. (1976). Antibody-dependent cell-mediated (K cell) cytotoxicity against isolated hepatocytes in chronic active hepatitis. *Lancet*, **1**, 441

Combes, B., Stastyny, P., Shorey, J., Eigenbrodt, E. H., Barrera, A., Hull, A. R. and Carter, N. W. (1971). Glomerulonephritis with deposition of Australia antigen–antibody complexes in glomerular basement membrane. *Lancet*, **2**, 234

Dawkins, R. L. and Joske, R. A. (1973). Immunoglobulin deposition in liver of patients with active chronic hepatitis and antibody against smooth muscle. *Br. Med. J.*, **2**, 643

Degast, G. C., Houwen, B. and Nieweg, H. O. (1973). Specific lymphocyte stimulation by purified, heat-inactivated hepatitis B antigen. *Br. Med. J.*, **4**, 707

Degast, G. C., Houwen, B., van der Hem, G. K. and The, T. H. (1976). T-lymphocyte number and function and the course of hepatitis B in hemodialysis patients. *Infect. Immun.*, **14**, 1138

De Horatius, R. J., Strickland, R. G. and Williams, R. C. (1974). T and B lymphocytes in acute and chronic hepatitis. *Clin. Immunol. Immunopath.*, **2**, 353

De Horatius, R. J., Henderson, C. and Strickland, R. G. (1976). Lymphocytotoxins in acute and chronic hepatitis: characterization and relationship to changes in circulating T lymphocytes. *Clin. Exp. Immunol.*, **26**, 21

Demura, M. C., Vernace, S. J. and Paronetto, F. (1975). Cell-mediated immune reactivity to hepatitis B surface antigen in liver disease. *Gastroenterology*, **69**, 310

Descamps, B., Jungers, P., Naret, C., Degott, C., Zingraff, J. and Bach, J. F. (1977). HLA-A₁, B₈-phenotype association and HBs antigenemia, evolution in 440 hemodialyzed patients. *Digestion*, **15**, 271

Doniach, D. (1970). The concept of an 'autoallergic' hepatitis. *Proc. Roy. Soc. Med.*, **63**, 527

Dudley, F. J., Fox, R. A. and Sherlock, S. (1972). Cellular immunity and hepatitis-associated Australia antigen liver disease. *Lancet*, **1**, 723

Endo, Y., Gudat, F., Bianchi, L., Mihatsch, N., Gasser, M., Stalder, G. A. and Schmid, M. (1978). Anti-HBc im Rahmen der Hepatitis-B-Virus Infektion: Korrelationen zu Entzündungsform und virusexpression. *Schweiz. Med. Wschr.*, **108**, 363

Farivar, M., Wands, J. R., Benson, G. D., Dienstag, J. L. and Isselbacher, K. J. (1976). Cryoprotein complexes and peripheral neuropathy in a patient with chronic active hepatitis. *Gastroenterology*, **71**, 490

Fernandez, R. and McCarthy, D. J. (1971). The arthritis of viral hepatitis. *Ann. Intern. Med.*, **74**, 207

POSSIBLE MECHANISMS OF TISSUE INJURY

Finlayson, N. D. C., Krohn, K., Fauconnet, M. H. and Anderson, K. E. (1972). Significance of serum complement levels in chronic liver disease. *Gastroenterology*, **63**, 653

Frei, P. C. Erard, P. and Zinkernagel, R. (1973). Cell-mediated immunity to hepatitis-associated antigen (HAA) demonstrated by leucocyte migration test during and after acute B hepatitis. *Biomedicine*, **19**, 379

Freudenberg, J., Baumann, H., Arnold, W., Berger, J. and Meyer zum Buschenfelde, K. H. (1977). HLA in different forms of chronic active hepatitis: a comparison between adult patients and children. *Digestion*, **15**, 260

Galbraith, R. M., Eddleston, A. L. W. F., Smith, M. G. M., Williams, R., Macsween, R. N. M., Watkinson, G., Dick, H., Kennedy, L. A. and Batchelor, J. R. (1974). Histocompatibility antigens in active chronic hepatitis and primary biliary cirrhosis. *Br. Med. J.*, **3**, 604

Galili, U., Eliakim, M., Slavin, S. and Schlesinger, M. (1975). Lymphocyte subpopulations in chronic active hepatitis: increase in lymphocytes forming stable E-rosettes. *Clin. Immunol. Immunopath.*, **4**, 538

Gerber, M. A., Brodin, A., Steinberg, D., Vernace, S., Yang, C. P. and Paronetto, F. (1972). Periarteritis nodosa, Australia antigen and lymphocytic leukemia. *N. Engl. J. Med.*, **286**, 14

Gerber, M. J., Phuangsab, A., Vittal, S. B. V., Dourdourekas, D., Steigmann, F. and Clowdus, B. F. (1974). Cell-mediated immune response to hepatitis B antigen in patients with liver disease. *Am. J. Digest. Dis.*, **19**, 637

Geubel, A. P., Keller, R. H., Summerskill, W. H. J., Dickson, E. R., Tomasi, T. B. and Shorter, R. G. (1976). Lymphocyte cytotoxicity and inhibition studied with autologous liver cells: observations in chronic active liver disease and the primary biliary cirrhosis syndrome. *Gastroenterology*, **71**, 450

Giantotti, F. (1973). Papular acrodermatitis of childhood: an Australia antigen disease. *Arch. Dis. Child.*, **48**, 794

Gocke, D. J., Hsu, K., Morgan, C., Bombardieri, S., Lockshin, M. and Christian, C. L. (1970). Association between polyarteritis and Australia antigen. *Lancet*, **2**, 1149

Hadzyannis, S. J. and Karvountzis, G. G. (1976). Serum anti-HBc titers in chronic liver disease. *Digestion*, **14**, 460

Heathcote, E. J., Dudley, F. J. and Sherlock, S. (1972). The association of polyarteritis and Australia antigen. *Digestion*, **6**, 280

Henson, P. M. (1971). Release of biologically active constituents from blood cells and its role in antibody-mediated tissue injury. In B. Amos (ed.) *Progress in Immunology*, p. 155 (New York: Academic Press)

Hillis, W. D., Hillis, A., Bias, W. B. and Walker, W. G. (1977). Associations of hepatitis B surface antigenemia with HLA locus B specificities. *N. Engl. J. Med.*, **296**, 1310

Hoofnagle, J. H., Gerety, R. J. and Barker, L. F. (1973). Antibody to hepatitis B virus core in man. *Lancet*, **2**, 869

Hoofnagle, J. H., Gerety, R. J., Ni, L. Y. and Barker, L. F. (1974). Antibody to hepatitis B core antigen, a sensitive indicator of persistent viral replication. *N. Engl. J. Med.*, **290**, 1336

Hoofnagle, J. H., Gerety, R. J. and Barker, L. F. (1975). Antibody to hepatitis B core antigen. *Am. J. Med. Sci.*, **270**, 179

Hopf, U., Meyer zum Buschenfelde, K. H. and Freudenberg, J. (1974). Liver specific antigens of different species. II. Localization of a membrane antigen at cell surface of isolated hepatocytes. *Clin. Exp. Immunol.*, **16**, 117

Hopf, U., Meyer zum Buschenfelde, K. H. and Arnold, W. (1976). Detection of a liver membrane autoantibody in HB-negative chronic active hepatitis. *N. Engl. J. Med.*, **294**, 572

Husby, G., Strickland, R. G., Caldwell, J. L. and Williams, R. C. (1975). Localization of T and B cells and α-fetoprotein in hepatic biopsies from patients with liver disease. *J. Clin. Invest.*, **56**, 1198

Irwin, G. R., Hierholzer, W. J., Cimis, R. and McCollum, R. W. (1974). Delayed hypersensitivity in hepatitis B: clinical correlates of in vitro production of migration inhibition factor. *J. Inf. Dis.*, **130**, 580

Ishimaru, H., Ito, K., Nakagawa, J. and Fukase, M. (1976). T cells and B cells in HBsAg-positive patients with chronic persistent hepatitis and asymptomatic carriers. *Ann. Inter. Med.*, **84**, 444

Joske, R. A., Turner, K. J. and Murphy, B. P. (1976). Serum IgE levels in patients with liver disease. *Med. J. Austr.*, **2**, 555

Jungers, P., Descamps, B., Zingraff, J., Naret, C. and Bach, J. F. (1975). Sur une corrélation entre les antigènes d'histocompatibilité HL-A 1 et 8 et une meilleure défense de l'urémique chronique contre le virus de l'hépatite. *C. R. Acad. Sci. (Paris)*, **281**, 675

Kawanishi, H. (1977). *In vitro* studies on IgG-mediated lymphocyte cytotoxicity in chronic active liver disease. *Gastroenterology*, **73**, 549

Kohler, P. F., Trembath, J., Merrill, D. A., Singleton, J. W. and Dubois, R. S. (1974). Immunotherapy with antibody, lymphocytes and transfer factor in chronic hepatitis B. *Clin. Immunol. Immunopath.*, **2**, 465

Krugman, S., Hoofnagle, J. H., Gerety, R. J., Kaplan, P. M. and Gerin, J. L. (1974). Viral hepatitis type B: DNA polymerase activity and antibody to hepatitis B core antigen. *N. Engl. J. Med.*, **290**, 1331

Kurokawa, S. (1976). A study on tissue mast cells in liver diseases. *Jap. J. Gastroenterol.*, **73**, 226

Laiwah, A. A. C. Y., Chaudhuri, A. K. R. and Anderson, J. R. (1973). Lymphocyte transformation and leukocyte migration-inhibition by Australia antigen. *Clin. Exp. Immunol.*, **25**, 27

Levo, Y., Gorevic, P. D., Kassab, H. J., Zucker-Franklin, D. and Franklin, E. C. (1977). Association between hepatitis B virus and essential mixed cryoglobulinemia. *N. Engl. J. Med.*, **296**, 1501

Mackey, I. R. and Morris, P. J. (1972). Association of autoimmune active chronic hepatitis with HL-A $_{1.8}$ *Lancet*, **2**, 793

Marner, I. L. (1952). The relation between hepatitis and polyarthritis. In *Rheumatic Diseases*, pp. 237–239 (Philadelphia: W. B. Saunders Company)

McIntosh, R. M., Koss, M. N. and Gocke, D. J. (1976). The nature and incidence of cryoproteins in hepatitis B antigen (HBsAg) positive patients. *Quat. J. Med.*, **45**, 23

Meyer zum Buschenfelde, K. H. and Miescher, P. A. (1972). Liver specific antigens. Purification and characterization. *Clin. Exp. Immunol.*, **10**, 89

Meyer zum Buschenfelde, K. H., Kossling, F. K. and Miescher, P. A. (1972). Experimental chronic active hepatitis in rabbits following immunization with human liver proteins. *Clin. Exp. Immunol.*, **10**, 99

Mikulski, S. M. (1976). K-cell function in patients with chronic aggressive hepatitis. *Lancet*, **2**, 44

Miller, D. J., Dwyer, J. M, and Klatskin, G. (1977). Identification of lymphocytes in percutaneous liver biopsy cores: Different T:B cell ratio in HBsAg-positive and -negative hepatitis. *Gastroenterology*, **72**, 1199

Newble, D. I., Holmes, K. T., Wangel, A. G. and Forbes, I. J. (1975). Immune reactions in acute viral hepatitis. *Clin. Exp. Immunol.*, **20**, 17

Ng, P. L., Powell, L. W. and Campbell, C. B. (1975). Guillain Barré syndrome during the pre-icteric phase of acute type B viral hepatitis. *Aust. N.Z. J. Med.*, **5**, 367

Onion, D. K., Crumpacker, C. S. and Gilliland, B. C. (1971). Arthritis of hepatitis associated with Australia antigen. *Ann. Intern. Med.*, **75**, 29

Paronetto. F. (1973). Immunologic aspect of liver disease. *Postgrad. Med.*, **53**, 156

Paronetto, F., Gerber, M. A. and Vernace, S. J. (1973). Immunologic studies in patients with chronic active hepatitis and primary biliary cirrhosis. 1. Cytotoxicity activity and binding of sera to human liver cells grown in tissue culture. *Proc. Soc. Exp. Biol. (NY)*, **143**, 756

Paronetto, F. and Vernace, S. (1975). Immunological studies in patients with chronic active hepatitis. Cytotoxic activity of lymphocytes to autochthonous liver cells grown in tissue culture. *Clin. Exp. Immunol.*, **19**, 99

Pettigrew, N. M., Goudie, R. B., Russell, R. I. and Chaudhuri, A. K. R. (1972). Evidence for a role of hepatitis virus B in chronic alcoholic liver disease. *Lancet*, **2**, 724

Prince, A. M. and Trepo, C. (1971). Role of immune complexes involving SH antigen in pathogenesis of chronic active hepatitis and polyarteritis nodosa. *Lancet*, **1**, 1309

Ray, M. B., Desmet, V. J., Bradburne, A. F., Desmyter, J., Fevery, J. and De Groote, J. (1976). Differential distribution of hepatitis B surface antigen and hepatitis B core antigen in the liver of hepatitis B patient. *Gastroenterology*, **71**, 462

Reed, W. D., Eddleston, A. L. W. F., Cullens, H., Williams, R., Zuckerman, A. J., Peters, D. K., Williams, D. G. and Maycock, W. A. (1973). Infusion of hepatitis B antibody in antigen positive active chronic hepatitis. *Lancet*, **2**, 1347

Review by an International Group (1977). Acute and chronic hepatitis revisited. *Lancet*, **2**, 914

Sanchez-Tapias, J., Thomas. H. C. and Sherlock, S. (1977). Lymphocyte populations in liver biopsy specimens from patients with chronic liver disease. *Gut*, **18**, 472

Sato, T., Arai, S., Nakamura, S. and Takezawa, Y. (1976). Phytohemagglutinin-induced lymphocyte transformation in liver diseases and in asymptomatic HBsAg carriers. *Tohoku J. Exp. Med.*, **118**, 99

Sergent, J. S., Lockshin, M. D., Christian, C. L. and Gocke, D. J. (1976). Vasculitis with hepatitis B antigenemia: Long term observation in nine patients. *Medicine*, **55**, 1

Sodomann, C. P., Havemann, K. and Martini, G. A. (1974). Cellular immune reactions in the course of virus hepatitis. *Digestion*, **10**, 328

Tage-Jensen, U., Arnold, W., Dietrichson, O., Hardt, F., Hopf, U., Meyer zum Buschenfelde, K. H. and Nielsen, J. O. (1977). Liver-cell-membrane autoantibody specific for inflammatory liver diseases. *Br. Med. J.*, **1**, 206

Thestrup-Pedersen, K., Ladefoged, K. and Andersen, P. (1976). Lymphocyte transformation test with liver specific protein and phytohaemagglutinin in patients with liver disease. *Clin. Exp. Immunol.*, **24**, 1

Thomson, A. D., Cochrane, M. A. G., McFarlane, I. G., Eddleston, A. L. W. F. and Williams, R. (1974). Lymphocyte cytotoxicity to isolated hepatocytes in chronic active hepatitis. *Nature*, **252**, 721

Thomas, H. C., Freni, M., Sanchez-Tapias, J., De Villiers, D., Jain, S. and Sherlock, S. (1976). Peripheral blood lymphocyte populations in chronic liver disease. *Clin. Exp. Immunol.*, **26**, 222

Toh, B. H., Roberts-Thomson, I. C., Mathews, J. D., Whittingham, S. and Mackay, I. R (1973). Depression of cell-mediated immunity in old age and the immunopathic diseases, lupus erythematosus, chronic hepatitis and rheumatoid arthritis. *Clin. Exp. Immunol.*, **14**, 193

Tolentino, P., Pasino, M., Braito, A., Astaldi, A. and Giacchino, R. (1974). Impaired T-lymphocyte function in chronic hepatitis. *Digestion*, **10**, 331

Trepo, C. G. and Thivolet, J. (1970). Hepatitis associated antigen and periarteritis nodosa (PAN). *Vox Sang. (Basel)*, **19**, 410

Trepo, C. G., Zuckerman, A. J., Bird, R. C. and Prince, A. M. (1974). The role of circulating hepatitis B antigen–antibody immune complexes in the pathogenesis of vascular and hepatic manifestations in polyarteritis nodosa. *J. Clin. Path.*, **27**, 863

Trepo, C. G., Robert, D., Motin, J., Trepo, D., Sepetjian, M. and Prince, A. M. (1976). Hepatitis B antigen (HBAg) and/or antibodies (anti-HBs; anti-HBc) in fulminant hepatitis. Pathogenic and prognostic significans. *Gut*, **17**, 10

Van Epps, D. E., Strickland, R. G. and Williams, R. C. (1975). Elevated IgE levels in liver disease. *Clin. Res.*, **23**, 106A

Wands, J. R. and Isselbacher, K. J. (1975). Lymphocyte cytotoxicity to autologous liver cells in chronic active hepatitis. *Proc. Natl. Acad. Sci. (USA)*, **72**, 1301

Wands, J. R., Mann, E., Alpert, E. and Isselbacher, K. J. (1975). The pathogenesis of arthritis associated with acute hepatitis B surface antigen-positive hepatitis. *J. Clin. Invest.*, **55**, 930

Warnatz, H. (1974). Immune reactions to hepatitis B antigen in acute and chronic hepatitis. *Acta Hepato-Gastroenterol.*, **21**, 237

Wicks, R. C., Kohler, P. R. and Singleton, J. W. (1975). Thymus-derived lymphocytes in type B acute viral hepatitis and healthy carriers of hepatitis B surface antigen (HBsAg). *Am. J. Dig. Dis.*, **20**, 518

Woolf, I. L., El Sheikh, N., Cullens, H., Lee, M. W., Eddleston, A. L. W. F., Williams, R. and Zuckerman. A. J. (1976). Enhanced HBsAb production in pathogenesis of fulminant viral hepatitis type B. *Br. Med. J.*, **2**, 669

Wright, R. (1970). The Australia antigen in chronic active hepatitis. *Vox. Sang.*, **19**, 320

11
Bidirectional immune attack in the pathogenesis of hepatitis B – an hypothesis

INTRODUCTION

As the pathogenesis of hepatitis B is still unknown, it has inevitably become a subject of frequent hypotheses (Dudley *et al.*, 1972; Popper and Mackay, 1972; Eddlestone and Williams, 1974; Edginton and Chisari, 1975). An increasing amount of evidence points to the important role of immune mechanisms in the development of the various histological types of hepatitis B. The topics of hepatitis B as well as immunological tissue injury are relatively new and developed during the same period. Information on these fields is still incomplete and fragmentary.

The present chapter deals with a hypothesis which is based on the synthesis of the results described in the previous chapters and is supported by relevant informations now available in this field.

The following series of facts will serve as premises to formulate the hypothesis.

(1) The two recognized distinct components of HBV – HBsAg and HBcAg – are identified by their respective antibodies. HBsAg is demonstrated in the cytoplasm and/or cell membrane of the hepatocytes. HBcAg is localized in the nucleus, the cytoplasm, and at the liver cell membrane (Ray *et al.*, 1976; Gudat and Bianchi, 1977).

(2) A diverse set of features is seen on histological examination of liver following HBV infections. The whole spectrum of liver morphology can be divided into three broad groups: *Non-aggressive group* – near normal liver, chronic persistent hepatitis and nonactive cirrhosis;

Aggressive group – chronic aggressive hepatitis, active cirrhosis and acute hepatitis with signs of transition to chronicity. The third group consists of *acute hepatitis* in its various developmental stages.

(3) The intrahepatic expressions of HBsAg and HBcAg are distinctive and correlate with the histological classification of hepatitis used in this book (Chapters 3 and 4).

There exists an inverse relation between the extent of liver cell necrosis and the amount of HBsAg in the liver. A huge amount of cytoplasmic HBsAg is observed in the non-aggressive group with absence or scanty presence of HBcAg. On the other hand membrane localized HBsAg with partial cytoplasmic positivity together with abundant HBcAg are characteristic of the aggressive group of hepatitis. In acute hepatitis, HBsAg as well as HBcAg is rarely demonstrable.

(4) As in fully developed acute hepatitis, HBV antigens are rarely demonstrated in the acute exacerbation of chronic aggressive hepatitis and in active cirrhosis.

(5) Cell membrane localized HBsAg has been demonstrated in isolated hepatocytes and in liver biopsies obtained in the prodromal stage of acute hepatitis B in chimpanzees and in humans (Chapter 7) (Alberti *et al.*, 1976).

(6) IgG with anti-HBc specificity is localized in HBcAg positive hepatocytes. *In vitro* complement fixation is demonstrated in the same liver cells suggesting intracellular formation of HBcAg immune complexes. Immune complexes with HBsAg specificity are not observed in HBsAg positive liver specimens.

(7) The presence of intrahepatocytic HBcAg immune complexes has been correlated with the histological pattern of disease. Such immune complexes are either absent or rarely demonstrable in non-aggressive hepatitis and in acute hepatitis.

(8) Our preliminary results show that absence of intrahepatic VCF and IgG and significant low titres of circulating anti-HBc in HBcAg positive patients are associated with minimal liver histological change.

(9) An HBsAg positive agammaglobulinaemic patient without circulating anti-HBc is associated with minimal liver damage (Chadwic *et al.*, 1978) whereas an hypogammaglobulinaemic patient is found to have chronic aggressive hepatitis (Tong *et al.*, 1977).

(10) Anti-HBs is detected much less frequently in the serum than anti-HBc, even when tested by a sensitive technique such as RIA. Anti-HBs is frequently detected in the convalescent stage of acute hepatitis B after the disappearnce of the antigen.

(11) Studies on serial serum samples during the developmental stages of hepatitis B in humans (Hoofnagle *et al.*, 1975) and in chimpanzees (Chapter 7) have clearly indicated that anti-HBc appears in the blood just prior to or at the onset of clinical hepatitis. Signs of hepatocytic damage also coincide with the formation of presumed intrahepatic HBcAg immune complexes in the chimpanzee suggesting that such immune complexes may be cytopathic.

(12) Infusion of serum containing high titres of anti-HBs in patients with HBsAg positive chronic aggressive hepatitis (Reed *et al.*, 1973) or in HBsAg positive chimpanzees (Trepo, 1975) fails to produce signs of liver damage.

(13) HBsAg immune complexes have been incriminated in the pathogenesis of extrahepatic abnormalities in hepatitis B.

(14) Opinions are almost equally divided on the precise identity and role of the aggressor lymhocytes in causing hepatocytic damage. Recent data on HBsAg positive chronic hepatitis show depression of T lymphocytes in the peripheral blood and an increase of such cells in the liver.

(15) Lymphocyte cytotoxicity on target cells (hepatocytes) has been claimed to be produced by T cells as well as K cells.

(16) By electron microscopy, lymphocytes have been demonstrated in close apposition with degraded hepatocytes in HBsAg positive chronic aggressive hepatitis (Kawanashi, 1977; Karasawa and Shikata, 1977). Some of the above points are summarized in Figure 11.1.

HYPOTHESIS: BIDIRECTIONAL IMMUNE ATTACK IN THE PATHOGENESIS OF HEPATITIS B

This hypothesis suggests that host immune mechanisms produced by HBV antigens cause liver cell necrosis and that HBV itself is not cytopathic. Liver cell injury may occur by two mechanisms: the surface phase (S-phase) and core phase (C-phase). For the initiation of the S-phase it is mandatory for HBsAg to be expressed in the cell membrane. In the C-phase the HBcAg has to be present not only in the hepatocytic nucleus but also in the cell cytoplasm and cell membrane. The S-phase is T or K cell dependent,

HEPATITIS B VIRUS ANTIGENS IN TISSUES

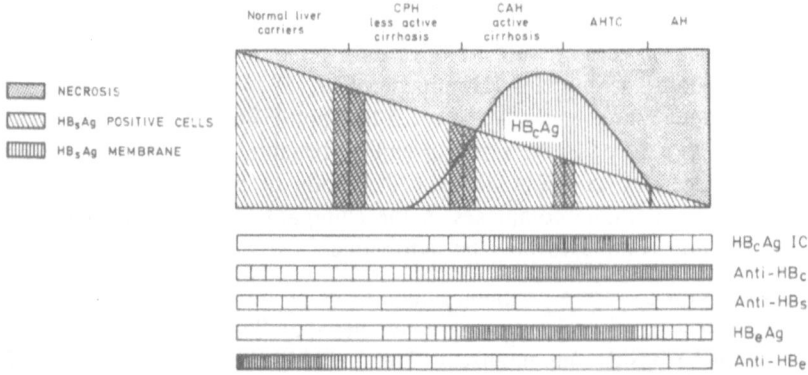

EXPRESSION OF HBV COMPONENTS
IN RELATION TO HEPATOCELLULAR NECROSIS

Figure 11.1 Diagramatic representation of the various hepatitis B virus associated markers in liver and in blood in hepatitis B

i.e. is mediated by aggressor lymphocytes. The C-phase is mediated by the intrahepatic deposition of HBcAg immune complexes. S and C-phases are operative simultaneously or independently. Liver cell necrosis will only occur when the intensity of specific immune reactions (i.e. cellular or immune complex) exceeds the threshold of tolerance of the hepatocytes. S-phase operates predominantly by causing liver cell damage of the 'piecemeal necrosis' type (Review, 1977) commonly observed in the aggressive group of chronic hepatitis. The C-phase is involved mostly in confluent liver cell necrosis, typically observed in fully developed acute hepatitis and in acute exacerbation of chronic hepatitis. The hypothetical role of S and C mechanisms in the causation of different types of liver cell necrosis is summarized in Table 11.1.

Table 11.1 Summary of the hypothetical role of S and C mechanisms in liver cell damage

Surface phase: S-phase	(1) HBsAg should be present in the cell membrane
	(2) T or K cell dependent
	(3) Causes periportal piecemeal necrosis
Core phase: C-phase	(1) HBcAg should be present in the cell membrane
	(2) Immune complexes dependent
	(3) Causes confluent liver cell necrosis

Immune mechanisms in acute hepatitis B

In the fully developed stage of acute hepatitis B, HBV antigens are rarely demonstrated in the liver most probably due to elimination of antigen-containing cells (Gudat *et al.*, 1975). However, both HBsAg and HBcAg are present in the early stage of acute hepatitis (Chapter 7).

In this situation predominantly the C-phase operates. HBcAg immune complexes have been observed in serial liver biopsies obtained during the developmental stages of acute hepatitis B. This has been found to coincide with the appearance of circulating anti-HBc and the onset of clinical hepatitis (Chapter 7).

Cell membrane expression of HBsAg in the prodromal stage may render the hepatocytes vulnerable to immune attack by sensitized lymphocytes (either T or K cells) which eventually produce cytolysis. The appearance of leukocyte migration inhibition by HBsAg (Dudley *et al.*, 1972; Demura *et al.*, 1975; Ibrahim *et al.*, 1975) may suggest the initiation of S-phase in acute hepatitis B. In the experimental studies on chimpanzees (Chapter 7), often single liver cells or groups of hepatocytes have been found to be surrounded or replaced by a group of mononuclear cells representing spotty liver cell necrosis.

In the later stages of acute hepatitis (resolving phase) membrane-localized HBsAg and HBcAg immune complexes are no longer demonstrable, indicating a decline of both the S and C-phase and allowing new cells to replace completely the damaged hepatocytes.

This mechanism of disappearance of HBV antigens from the hepatocytes is not the only working hypothesis. In 1975, Edgington and Chisari (1975) suggested that the clearance of the HBV may be the result of immunological suppression rather than elimination of the infected hepatocytes.

Immune mechanisms in chronic hepatitis B

In chronic hepatitis B including active cirrhosis and acute hepatitis with signs of transition to chronicity, both the S and C-phases operate. The S-phase may be predominant as there is abundant membrane expression of HBsAg. Aggressor lymphocytes accumulate in the portal fields and come in close contact with periportal hepatocytes. Cell damage occurs by direct cytotoxicity or indirectly through the release of lymphokines. Recently mononuclear cells have been observed in direct apposition with the hepatocytes in HBsAg positive chronic aggressive hepatitis (Kawanishi, 1977; Karasawa and Shikata, 1977). Such a mechanism in liver cell death has been suggested previously (Dudley *et al.*, 1972).

The rate of cell death in S-phase is apparently slow, and may be due to inadequate sensitization or genetic deficiency of the aggressor lymphocytes. Membrane-localized HBsAg has been demonstrated in repeated liver biopsies obtained from the same patients at different periods of time (unpublished data). A continuous process of cell death and eventual replacement by newly reinfected cells may explain this observation.

The participation of the C-phase in chronic hepatitis B is facultative. HBcAg immune complexes have been demonstrated in relatively high amounts in HBcAg positive hepatocytes. *In vivo* complement fixation has not been demonstrated but IgG has been visualized only in HBcAg positive specimens. In this condition, since a high number of hepatocytes are still present, HBcAg immune complexes as such cannot be held responsible for cell death. Nevertheless, it may be speculated that these complexes induce cytolysis when the complement system is also transported and activated inside the cells. Cytolysis should be rapid in this case, since *in vivo* complement fixation has not been visualized. The C-phase apparently only starts when a group of hepatocytes is optimally loaded with HBcAg immune complexes. Cell necrosis will be rapid and may lead to confluent necrosis. This phenomenon is usually seen in the acute exacerbation stage in chronic hepatitis B.

In healthy HBsAg carriers, both membrane-localized HBsAg and HBcAg immune complexes are absent. S and C-phase cannot be initiated, therefore liver cell necrosis is minimal or absent in these cases.

In this system the role of HBsAg immune complexes in the development of hepatitis B has been given least consideration because of the obvious difficulty in demonstrating circulating anti-HBs in the presence of HBsAg. There are only isolated reports on the presence of anti-HBs in the early stage of acute hepatitis B (Woolf *et al.*, 1976; Trepo *et al.*, 1976). However, circulating anti-HBs is fairly common in the later stage of acute hepatitis in absence of HBsAg. Moreover the presence of anti-HBs immune complexes could not be correlated with hepatocellular damage (Reed *et al.*, 1973; Trepo, 1975; Wright and Rassam, 1976). In contrast to the lack of evidence for a causative role of HBsAg immune complexes in the development of hepatitis B, such immune complexes have been implicated in the pathogenesis of extrahepatic diseases (Chapter 9 and 10). In these locations the complexes are sequestrated in special structures (e.g. glomerular basement membrane) where immune damage may be more compatible with prolonged cellular survival than in HBsAg-producing hepatocytes.

Table 11.2 summarizes the mechanism of tissue damage in HBV infection according to the present hypothesis. Liver damage is produced by host immune mechanisms against HBsAg which act through type IV and/or type V reactions and HBcAg which acts through type III reactions. Extra-

Table 11.2

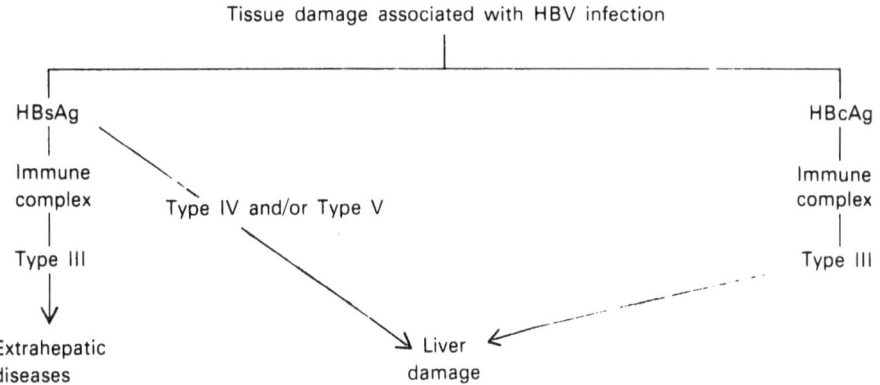

hepatic tissue damage is caused by deposition of HBsAg immune complexes (type III reactions).

In summary: HBsAg is related to cell mediated immune attack, while HBcAg is related to humoral immune mechanisms.

References

Alberti, A., Realdi, G., Tremolada, F. and Spina, G. P. (1976). Liver cell surface localization of hepatitis B antigen and of immunoglobulins in acute and chronic hepatitis and in liver cirrhosis. *Clin. Exp. Immunol.*, **25**, 396

Chadwic, R. G., Thomas, H. C. and Sherlock, S. (1978). e-Antigen in agammaglobinaemia *Lancet*, **1**, 617

Demura, M. C., Vernace, S. J. and Paronetto, F. (1975). Cell mediated immune reactivity to hepatitis B surface antigen in liver disease. *Gastroenterology*, **69**, 310

Dudley, F. J., Fox, R. A. and Sherlock, S. (1972). Cellular immunity and hepatitis associated. Australia antigen liver disease. *Lancet*, **1**, 723

Eddlestone, A. L. W. F. and Williams, R. (1974). Inadequate antibody response to HBAg or suppressor T-cell defect in development of active chronic hepatitis. *Lancet*, **2**, 1543

Edgington, T. S. and Chisari, F. V. (1975). Immunological aspects of hepatitis B virus infection. *Am. J. Med. Sci.*, **270**, 213

Gudat, F., Bianchi, L., Sonnabend, W., Thiel, G., Aenishaenslin, W. and Stalder, G. A. (1975). Pattern of core and surface expression in liver tissue reflects state of specific immune response in hepatitis. *Lab. Invest.*, **32**, 1

Gudat, F. and Bianchi, L. (1977). Evidence for phasic sequences in nuclear HBcAg formation and cell membrane directed flow of core particles in chronic hepatitis B. *Gastroenterology*, **73**, 1194

Hoofnagle, J. H., Gerety, R. J. and Barker, L. F. (1975). Antibody to hepatitis B core antigen. *Am. J. Med. Sci.*, **270**, 179

Ibrahim, A. B., Vyas, G. N. and Perkins, H. A. (1975). Immune response to hepatitis B surface antigen. *Infect. Immun.*, **11**, 137

Karasawa, T. and Shikata, T. (1977). Necrosis of the hepatocytes with hepatitis B surface antigen. *Arch. Path.*, **101**, 280

Kawanishi, H. (1977). Morphologic association of lymphocytes with hepatocytes in chronic liver disease. *Arch. Path.*, **101**, 286

Popper, H. and Mackay, I. R. (1972). Relation between Australian antigen and auto-immune hepatitis. *Lancet*, **1**, 1161

Ray, M. B., Desmet, V. J., Bradburne, A. F., Desmyter, J., Fevery, J. and De Groote, J. (1976). Differential distribution of hepatitis B surface antigen and hepatitis B core antigen in the liver of hepatitis B patients. *Gastroenterology*, **71**, 462

Reed, W. D., Eddleston, A. L. W. F., Cullens, H., Williams, R., Zuckerman, A. J., Peters, D. K., William, D. G. and May, W. A. (1973). Infusion of hepatitis B antibody in antigen positive active chronic hepatitis. *Lancet*, **2**, 1347

Review by an International Group (1977). Acute and chronic hepatitis revisited. *Lancet*, **2**, 914

Tong, M., Nies, K. M. and Redeker, A. (1977). Rapid progression of chronic active type B hepatitis in a patient with hypogammaglobulinemia. *Gastroenterology*, **73**, 1418

Trepo, C. G. (1975). Viral hepatitis; immune mechanisms. Discussion. *Am. J. Med. Sci.*, **270**, 248

Trepo, C. G., Robert, D., Motin, J., Trepo, D., Sepetjian, M. and Prince, A. M. (1976). Hepatitis B antigen (HBAg) and /or antibodies (anti-HBs; anti-HBc) in fulminant hepatitis. Pathogenic and prognostic significans. *Gut*, **17**, 10

Woolf, I. L., el Sheikh, N., Cullens, H., Lee, M. W., Eddleston, A. L. W. F., Williams, R. and Zuckerman, A. J. (1976). Enhanced HBsAb production in pathogenesis of fulminant viral hepatitis type B. *Br. Med. J.*, **2**, 669

Wright, R. and Rassam, S. (1976). The immunology of acute and chronic hepatitis. *Clinics in Gastroenterology*, **5**, 387

Summary and general conclusions

Blumberg's incidental discovery of Australia antigen (HBsAg) and its association with hepatitis B has led to the characterization of hepatitis B virus (HBV). It is a circular double stranded (mol. wt. 1.6×10^6) DNA virus composed of at least two distinct antigens. The outer surface or envelop contains HBsAg, a non-nucleoprotein–phospholipid–carbohydrate complex, antigenically heterogeneous, having a group specific determinant 'a' and mutually exclusive subdeterminant pairs d–y and w–r. The 28 nm inner core contains core protein (HBcAg), viral specific DNA and DNA polymerase. HBeAg may be related to the virion (Dane particle).

Methods are now available to detect HBV components in the infected host. Chapter 1 deals with a description of the basic materials and procedures applied for detecting HBsAg and HBcAg in tissue sections and in blood. The results obtained with those procedures are evaluated in Chapter 2. For the demonstration of HBsAg in frozen sections, the modified fluorescence technique (heating test) has been shown to be superior to the conventional method; in paraffin sections, the specific immunohistochemical methods (immunofluorescence and PAP) are better than Shikata's modified orcein and routine haematoxylin–eosin (observation of ground glass hepatocytes) stainings. Nevertheless, the histological techniques are inexpensive and technically simple. HBsAg is localized in the cytoplasm and/or cell membrane of the hepatocytes whereas the immunofluorescence technique applied on frozen sections reveals HBcAg mostly in the hepatocytic nuclei and rarely in the cytoplasm and cell membrane. These findings are confirmed by the ultrastructural demonstration of HBsAg associated filaments and HBcAg associated core particles in the respective cellular sites.

Chapter 3 deals with the incidence and intrahepatic expression patterns of HBsAg in chronic hepatitis and in acute hepatitis. In chronic hepatitis, HBsAg is more prevalent in the liver (68%) than in the blood (57%) whereas a reverse situation is present in the case of acute hepatitis (50% in serum;

33% in liver). The distinctive intrahepatic distribution of HBsAg correlates with the histological classification of hepatitis. Membrane-localized HBsAg, which is observed predominantly in aggressive forms of chronic hepatitis B, has also been directly correlated with the presence of HBcAg in the hepatocytes (Chapter 4). Abundant intrahepatic accumulation of HBcAg is observed in patients treated with immunosuppressive drugs in contrast to its absence in cases in the fully developed stage of acute hepatitis and in the acute exacerbation stage of chronic hepatitis. In chronic hepatitis, the presence of membrane-localized HBsAg and nuclear HBcAg is also correlated with the demonstration of *in vitro* complement fixation (VCF) and immunoglobulin deposition in the liver specimens (Chapter 5). Based on this correlation, a suggestion has been made of the usefulness of these parameters in differentiating aggressive from non-aggressive forms of hepatitis B. Further, as VCF has only been observed in cases with intrahepatic HBcAg along with circulating anti-HBc but not with anti-HBs, it is postulated that intrahepatic deposition of HBcAg immune complexes may cause hepatocytic damage.

Chapter 6 deals with the demonstration of HBsAg in 44 cases of hepatocellular carcinoma. Forty-three per cent are positive, among which 84% are cirrhotic. Cytoplasmic HBsAg is abundant and more frequent in non-hepatoma cells compared with that observed in hepatoma cells. HBsAg, although in small amounts, is more readily detectable in moderately than in poorly differentiated hepatocellular carcinoma.

The experimental induction of hepatitis B (Chapter 7) is an investigation essentially performed to explore sequentially the immunopathological events; this study is complementary to the study previously described by Barker and co-workers. Membrane-localized HBsAg is observed in the incubation stage but not in the later stage of resolving acute hepatitis. Intrahepatic HBcAg immune complexes are demonstrated at the onset of clinical hepatitis along with the appearance of circulating anti-HBc but not with anti-HBs. It is suggested, as far as the participation of immune mechanisms is concerned, that diverse host reactions to both HBsAg and HBcAg are probably the determining factors in producing hepatocytic damage.

In Chapter 8, the effect of human fibroblast interferon is investigated on three subjects (two chimpanzees and one patient) with chronic hepatitis B infection. Intramuscular injection of 10^7 IU of interferon over two weeks depresses profoundly the nucleocapsid hepatitis B core antigen in the liver, indicating that hepatitis B virus infection is sensitive to interferon. The results obtained are similar to those of the other two studies performed, using human leukocyte interferon and interferon inducer respectively. Although the effect of interferon is short lived, controlled and long term treatment may be more valuable in hepatitis B virus infection.

Hepatitis B virus infection is often associated with extrahepatic diseases. In the present investigation (Chapter 9) HBsAg is demonstrated in 42% of kidney biopsies with histologically diagnosed various types of glomerulo-nephritis. The highest incidence of positivity is obtained in the membranous type. The available liver biopsies show chronic hepatitis including cirrhosis. HBsAg immune complexes are demonstrated in the kidney but not in the liver, confirming previous observations mentioned in the text and suggesting that such immune complexes produce extrahepatic abnormalities without necessarily being pathogenic to the liver.

In Chapter 10, the actual state of knowledge of the possible mechanisms of tissue injury in hepatitis B virus infection is discussed systematically. The information available suggests that the host's immunological reactions to the hepatitis B virus antigens rather than HBV itself are cytopathic. Although sensitized lymphocytes are found to be hepatocytotoxic, the precise identity and role of these aggressor cells remain unknown. HBsAg immune complexes have been found to produce extrahepatic tissue injury but circumstantial evidence militates against the role of such immune complexes in hepatocellular damage. On the other hand the potential hepatocytopathic effect of HBcAg immune complexes cannot be excluded. Genetic factors most probably control both cellular and humoral immunity and subsequent development of chronic hepatitis. Based on the gathered observations and available information, the last chapter (Chapter 11) deals with a working hypothesis which suggests that liver damage is produced by HBsAg acting through type IV and/or type V host immune reactions and by HBcAg acting through type III reactions. Extrahepatic tissue injury is initiated by the deposition of HBsAg immune complexes (type III reaction).

Index

DAB *see* diaminobenzene
Dane particles 5, 42, 45, 109, 116, 128
   see also HBsAg
  assembly 75
  in CAH sera 75
diaminobenzene (DAB) 31
Disse's space 42
DNA
  in HBV core 6, 157
  polymerase 7, 157
drugs, immunosuppressive 39, 40,
   70, 114
  and HBcAg positive nuclei 75
  and HBV antigen proportions 72, 73
  and lymphocyte toxicity 142

electron microscopy 41–6, 75
  immune 42, 45
  virus particle characterization,
   44, 157
endoplasmic reticulum
  Dane particles in 45
  smooth 38
enzyme immunoassay 17

FITC *see* fluorescein isothiocyanate
fluorescence microscopy 13
  compared with RIA 50, 51
  in glomerulonephritis 126
  of HBcAg 38–41, 75, 80, 81
  of HBsAg 23–8, 58–60, 92, 93, 96,
   105, 126
  of HCC liver 92, 93
fluorescein isothiocyanate (FITC)
  anti-HBc 80
  goat antirabbit- (GAR) 78
  rabbit antihuman- (RAHu) 78

gel diffusion 16
glomerulonephritis 88, 137, 139
  focal 125
  HBsAg demonstrated in patients
   123–9
  HBsAg induced 123
  immune complex deposition in 124
  intracapillary 125, 127
  membranoproliferative 125, 127
  membranous 125–7
Guillain Barré syndrome 137

haemagglutination inhibition 17
haemodialysis, and glomerulonephritis
  127
haemophilia lipoprotein antibody 3
haemotoxylin and eosin stain 36, 37
HBcAg *see* hepatitis B, core antigen
HBeAg *see* hepatitis B, e-antigen
HBsAg *see* hepatitis B, surface antigen
HBV *see* hepatitis B virus
HCC *see* hepatocellular carcinoma
hepatitis
  long incubation (MS$_2$) 4
  serum 4
  short incubation (MS$_1$) 4
hepatitis B
  active chronic 6
  acute 18, 51, 53, 62, 71, 117, 150
   and immune mechanisms 153
  acute with signs of chronicity
   (AHTC) 18, 50, 53, 83–5
   circulating antibodies in 81–4
   HBcAg distribution 74
   HBsAg distribution 63, 71, 74
  aggressive 150 *see also* CAH, AHTC
  anicteric 109

  chronic
   and HBsAg in liver 55
   HBsAg status effects 50, 53, 54
   and immune mechanisms 153–5
  chronic aggressive (CAH) 18, 34, 36,
   43, 50, 54, 82–5, 98, 116, 142
   antigen proportions in 72, 73
   anti-HBc titres 136
   HBsAg incidence 55, 57
   role of immunity 88
  chronic persistent (CPH) 18, 34, 53
   82–5, 98
   HBsAg incidence 55, 74
   HBsAg in liver 56–8
  core antigen (HBcAg) 5, 6, 77–88,
   151
   in active cirrhosis 85
   in acute hepatitis 71, 74, 82–4
   in AHTC 71, 74, 82
   assessment 69
   carriers 98
   in chronic hepatitis 71, 74, 80,
   82–5